Studies in Computational Intelligence

Volume 1230

The series "Studies in Computational Intelligence" (SCI) publishes new developments and advances in the various areas of computational intelligence—quickly and with a high quality. The intent is to cover the theory, applications, and design methods of computational intelligence, as embedded in the fields of engineering, computer science, physics and life sciences, as well as the methodologies behind them. The series contains monographs, lecture notes and edited volumes in computational intelligence spanning the areas of neural networks, connectionist systems, genetic algorithms, evolutionary computation, artificial intelligence, cellular automata, self-organizing systems, soft computing, fuzzy systems, and hybrid intelligent systems. Of particular value to both the contributors and the readership are the short publication timeframe and the world-wide distribution, which enable both wide and rapid dissemination of research output.

Indexed by SCOPUS, DBLP, WTI AG (Switzerland), zbMATH, SCImago.

All books published in the series are submitted for consideration in Web of Science.

KC Santosh · Debasmita Ghosh Roy

Artificial Intelligence for Human Fertility: Trends, Insights, and Predictions

Springer

KC Santosh
AI Research Laboratory, Department of Computer Science
University of South Dakota
Vermillion, SD, USA

Debasmita Ghosh Roy
School of Automation, Banasthali Vidyapith
Tonk, Rajasthan, India

ISSN 1860-949X ISSN 1860-9503 (electronic)
Studies in Computational Intelligence
ISBN 978-981-95-1247-8 ISBN 978-981-95-1248-5 (eBook)
https://doi.org/10.1007/978-981-95-1248-5

This Springer imprint is published by the registered company Springer Nature Singapore Pte Ltd.
The registered company address is: 152 Beach Road, #21-01/04 Gateway East, Singapore 189721, Singapore

Preface

The declining global Total Fertility Rate (TFR) is a critical issue impacting both developed and developing countries, with far-reaching effects on economic conditions. Common economic indicators such as GDP, HDI, and population metrics are often used to evaluate a country's status. This book studies/explores the reasons behind the dramatic decline in TFR, which has dropped to half of its previous levels. A major factor contributing to this trend is the widespread lack of recognition of fertility issues as a medical concern, compounded by insufficient societal awareness. To better understand the dynamics of human reproduction, this book identifies various factors that influence fertility, including the male and female reproductive systems, lifestyle choices, career demands, societal pressures, environmental factors, and personal habits (e.g. millennials).

Central to this understanding is the collection of vast amounts of data, for which AI algorithms play a crucial role. The book studies how AI can help predict fertility outcomes by analyzing diverse datasets for both male and female populations. It also discusses the growing reliance on Assisted Reproductive Technologies, despite their high costs and inconsistent success rates, and how AI can assist in predicting these success rates to ease the financial burden on patients. The primary goal of this book is to highlight how (explainable) AI can become a powerful tool in predicting human fertility. Ultimately, it aims at raising the global TFR and addressing the challenges posed by declining fertility rates around the world.

Vermillion, USA — KC Santosh
Tonk, India — Debasmita Ghosh Roy

Competing Interests The authors have no competing interests to declare that are relevant to the content of this manuscript.

Contents

About the Authors

Prof. KC Santosh, a highly accomplished AI Expert and TEDx Speaker, is the Chair of the Department of Computer Science (since 2020) and founding director of the AI Lab (since 2015, https://ai-reseach-lab.org) at the University of South Dakota (USD). He served as Graduate Program Director for seven years (2017–24) and was previously a research fellow at NIH and a PostDoc at INRIA (France). At USD, he has overseen five degree-granting programs, including six specializations and certificates, managed 15 faculty and three staff, supported ~ 500 students, and administered a budget of over $2.2 million, including research grants. With over $8.7 million in funding (DOD, NSF, and ED, to name a few), he has authored 11 books and 250+ research articles (such as IEEE TPAMI, IEEE TAI, and IEEE TMI). He serves as an associate editor for *IEEE Transactions on Artificial Intelligence, IEEE Transactions of Medical Imaging* and *International Journal of Machine Learning and Cybernetics* and leads review panels for NSF and Mitacs (Canada). He is a trained leader, having completed leadership programs such as Deans/Chairs 1.0 (CCAS, Spring 2021), Deans/Chairs 2.0 (CCAS, Summer 2024), and the President Executive Leadership Institute (USD, 2021/22). He leads the AI+X initiative that primarily includes curriculum innovation, the South Dakota Biomedical Computation Collaborative (supported by a $0.745 M award from the SD Board of Regents and a $6.5 M award from the U.S. Department of Education) and USD's IEEE-Sponsored AI symposium (since 2018). He brings extensive experience in curriculum innovation, particularly in interdisciplinary initiatives and shared governance (e.g. physics, business analytics, psychology, biology, biomedical engineering, etc.) as well as in program assessment and evaluation (as PEV), including ABET accreditation during the 2016/17 and 2022/23 cycles. His leadership has driven more than 3000% growth in AI enrollment at USD. His contributions have established USD as a pioneer in AI programs within the state of South Dakota. In fundraising, he secured a $2.0 million endowment to further strengthen the reputation of the department. He is a member of the NIST's AI Standards and Innovation (previously named as AI Safety Institute Consortium) and a U.S. Speaker for AI education. For more info. https://kc-santosh.org/.

Dr. Debasmita Ghosh Roy is an Assistant Professor at the School of Automation, Banasthali Vidyapith (BV). She received her B.Tech. in Applied Electronics and Instrumentation from the West Bengal University of Technology (WBUT), India, in 2008, and her M.Tech. in Control and Instrumentation from WBUT in 2012. Dr. Roy completed her Ph.D. in Control and Instrumentation (specialized in AI for human fertility assessment) from Banasthali Vidyapith, Rajasthan, India, in 2025. Her research interests include bioinformatics, pattern recognition, machine learning, deep learning, Explainable AI, and data analytics. She is a member of the AI Research Lab (https://ai-research-lab.org).

Abbreviations

ADA	Adaboost
ADASYN	Adaptive Synthetic Sampling
AI	Artificial Intelligence
AMH	Anti-Mullerian Hormone
ANNs	Artificial Neural Network
ART	Assisted Reproductive Techniques
ASFR	Age-Specific Fertility Rate
CBR	Crude Birth Rate
CBT	Catboost
CFS	Correlation-Based Feature Selection
CNNs	Convolution Neural Network
DL	Deep Learning
DT	Decision Tree
EHRs	Electronic Health Records
ENN	Edited Nearest Neighbors
FNN	Feedforward Neural Network
FSH	Follicle-Stimulating Hormone
GANs	Generative Adversarial Networks
GBT	Gradient Boost
GDP	Gross Domestic Product
HDI	The Human Development Index
HPG	Hypothalamic-Pituitary-Gonadal
ICA	Independent Component Analysis
IVF	In Vitro Fertilization
K-NN	K-Nearest Neighbor
KPCA	Kernel Principal Component Analysis
LDA	Linear Discriminant Analysis
LE	Laplacian Eigenmaps
LH	Luteinizing Hormone
LLE	Locally Linear Embedding
LR	Logistic Regression

MDS	Multidimensional Scaling
ML	Machine Learning
MLP	Multi-Layer Perceptron
NB	Naïve Bays
NCA	Neighborhood Component Analysis
NMF	Non-Negative Matrix Factorization
PCA	Principal Component Analysis
PCOS	Polycystic Ovarian Syndrome
PID	Pelvic Inflammatory Disease
RDF	Random Decision Forest
SMOTE	Synthetic Minority Over-Sampling Technique
SVD	Singular Value Decomposition
SVM	Support Vector Machine
TFR	Total Fertility Rate
T-sne	T-Distributed Stochastic Neighbor Embedding
WHO	World Health Organization
XGB	Extreme Gradient Boost

List of Figures

List of Tables

Chapter 1
Human Fertility and Global Trends

1.1 Introduction

Fertility is a natural capability encompassing gamete production, fertilization, and pregnancy. Over the past decades, the World Health Organization has noted a decline in fertility rates [1]. About 17.5% of adults, or approximately one in six individuals globally grapple, with infertility. Medical reports emphasize the individualized nature of this issue, reflecting its complexity, influenced by numerous factors. Despite the prevalence of infertility, many couples don't categorize it as a disease. Rather, they perceive it as an inherent physiological process rather than a pathological disorder. The diverse experiences couples encounter underscore the intricate landscape of fertility. While not all couples face challenges in conceiving, the absence of fertility or difficulties in achieving pregnancy does not necessarily equate to a diseased state [2]. The ongoing infertility crisis is indisputable, yet its subtlety lies in the fact that symptoms often remain inconspicuous without a thorough medical assessment. These concealed indicators emphasize the importance of proper medical evaluation to discern fertility-related concerns accurately.

It is important to acknowledge the evolving attitudes towards infertility across different regions. While many low and middle-income countries still grapple with high fertility rates due to limited access to contraception and family planning services, changes are taking place. This narrative is backed by clear evidence extensively documented in reputable journals [3–5]. Amid this context, a significant aspect of reproductive health that often remains overlooked globally is infertility or declining fertility rates [6]. Recent global data underline the magnitude of this issue, revealing that 48 million couples and 180 million individuals globally are impacted by infertility. This mounting global challenge has prompted international organizations, healthcare professionals, and patient advocacy groups to collaborate in offering support, information, and services for those affected by infertility. The aim is to address the immediate concerns and tackle the broader societal, economic, and healthcare implications it entails.

KC. Santosh and D. G. Roy, *Artificial Intelligence for Human Fertility: Trends, Insights, and Predictions*, Studies in Computational Intelligence 1230,
https://doi.org/10.1007/978-981-95-1248-5_1

Infertility finds its roots in physiological factors, but its consequences extend far beyond by presenting diverse impacts on individuals and couples [7]. The complex aftermath often manifests in mental and psychological well-being, with anxiety and depression emerging as frequent companions [8]. The emotional journey of trying to conceive and facing infertility challenges can be highly stressful. It evokes a range of emotions, including feelings of isolation, loneliness, diminished self-esteem, relationship strain, and negative thought patterns [9–11]. Additionally, infertility treatments further contribute to emotional distress, intensifying the psychological burden. These emotional factors can act as triggers, exacerbating the challenges associated with infertility. Consequently, seeking support and implementing coping mechanisms are crucial for managing mental health, influencing emotional well-being, and potentially affecting fertility outcomes. In this context, personalized support plays a vital role as couples undergo infertility treatments. It is essential to recognize that infertility treatment approaches are highly individualized, tailored to the unique circumstances of each case. Furthermore, the guidance of a reproductive specialist is essential in unravelling the foundational causes of infertility and crafting a bespoke treatment roadmap [12]. Infertility treatments impose demands that span the physical, emotional, and financial realms. Thus, fostering transparent communication between patients and physicians becomes indispensable for comprehensively understanding potential advantages, risks, and alternatives. The treatment protocols encompass a spectrum of medical interventions, with ARTs reigning as prevalent choices [13]. ART revolves around the technology harnessed for treating eggs, sperm, fertilized eggs, and embryos [14]. The groundwork for ART procedures entails meticulous evaluation and analysis to decode the underlying causes of infertility. This all-encompassing methodology entails elements like intracytoplasmic sperm injection, in vitro fertilization, cryopreservation of embryos or gametes, and the administration of associated medications. These intricate processes are marked by their time-intensive nature and often harbour an element of uncertainty. The effectiveness of ART treatments can exhibit variability due to a range of factors, and achieving success in every treatment cycle is not guaranteed. Multiple attempts might be required to achieve a successful pregnancy [15]. Hence, it is crucial not to overlook the emotional repercussions that influence success rates. Additionally, lifestyle and behavioural factors substantially influence fertility rates, and the eventual treatment outcome is closely intertwined with these factors [16].

Infertility trends within the millennial generation encompass a broad spectrum of individual experiences and choices, exemplifying diversity [17]. The dynamics of lifestyle have undergone substantial transformations in recent decades. Despite the presence of infertility cases in earlier eras, the sudden surge in its incidence presents an enigmatic scenario. Multiple sources emphasize the positive influence of healthy lifestyle choices on the human reproductive system. Conversely, an unhealthy lifestyle can hinder the prospects of both natural conception and successful outcomes through ART. In certain instances, infertility cases evade clear explication, falling under the idiopathic or unexplained infertility category, thus introducing an additional layer of concern. These unforeseen fluctuations in fertility patterns trigger apprehensions about underlying health factors. The linkage between various comorbidities and infertility also heightens concerns [18]. Among the prevalent comorbidities are cardiovascular disease, gynecologic malignancies, diabetes mellitus, hypertension, hyperthyroidism, autoimmune diseases, asthma, and psychiatric disorders [19–21].

Growing evidence shows that infertility affects both men and women. Many studies have explored how male and female infertility relate to clinical and lifestyle factors. Similarly, research has examined the link between infertility, reproductive disorders, and long-term health effects in both genders. In women's infertility, common conditions like PCOS and endometriosis often indicate potential future health risks [22]. In male infertility, hypertension is a common comorbidity, affecting seminal parameters and DNA fragmentation, both key biomarkers of fertility. Obesity is also a major factor, as a high BMI is closely linked to impaired spermatogenesis. Additionally, inflammatory arthritis and diabetes are associated with reduced overall reproductive health [23].

Infertility is classified into two types: primary (when a couple has never conceived) and secondary (when a couple struggles to conceive again after a previous successful pregnancy). In both cases, a thorough diagnostic evaluation is essential. Evidence suggests that age plays a crucial role as a key demographic factor influencing fertility. In women, egg quality and quantity decline with age, while men experience reductions in sperm count, motility, and morphology, leading to a higher proportion of abnormally shaped sperm. Several factors contribute to infertility, including diet and nutrient intake, alcohol consumption, smoking habits, sleep patterns, physical activity, caffeine intake, exposure to environmental toxins, pollutants, chemicals, sexual health, sexual frequency, and birth control use among women [24]. Among these, environmental toxins and occupational exposures are particularly challenging to modify, making proper guidance essential to minimize their impact. Hence, using flexible strategies can help manage these factors that affect and reduce the risk of unexplained infertility [25]. Despite infertility not being overlooked worldwide, the average number of births per woman is steeply declining. Figure 1.1 highlights the changing trends in birth rates since 1950. Projections reveal a steady decline in global fertility, averaging around 0.41% annually. This downward trend suggests that societies may be unprepared for the far-reaching consequences of declining birth rates [26].

1.2 Human Fertility and Global Dynamics

Global dynamics encompass the intricate interplay and interdependencies among diverse global regions. These dynamics yield avenues for collaborative advancement while presenting concurrent challenges. A comprehensive examination of various factors is imperative to grasp the correlation between human fertility and global dynamics. Thus, the relationship is multifaceted and encompasses influential aspects such as societal economic progress, education, empowerment, family planning, healthcare, environmental considerations, cultural and religious dimensions,

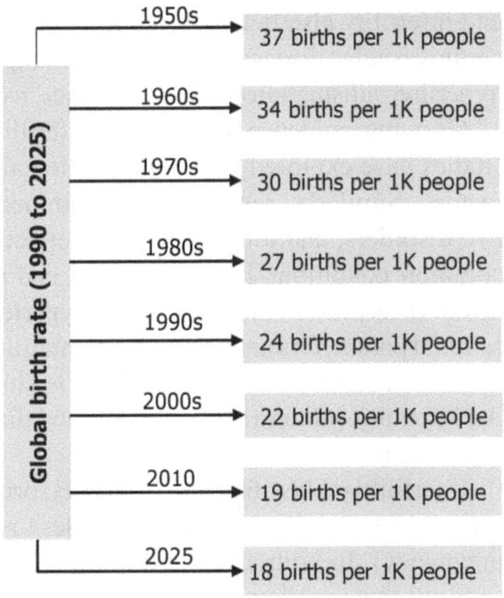

Fig. 1.1 Bar chart showing the decline in global birth rates from the 1950s to 2025. Each decade is labelled with the corresponding birth rate per 1000 people: 1950s (37), 1960s (34), 1970s (30), 1980s (27), 1990s (24), 2000s (22), 2010 (19), and 2025 (18). The chart highlights a consistent decrease over time

aging populations, and more [27]. Collectively, these factors shape global population growth and distribution. The major factors that are profound in human fertility are depicted in Fig. 1.2. Each of them will be described in the following sections.

Population growth

The rate of human fertility significantly influences the pace of population growth. The correlation between population growth and fertility rate is directly proportional, which makes the fertility rate a pivotal determinant of population dynamics. It signifies the average number of offspring born to women within a specific population and reproductive age range. A rate exceeding 2.1, while accounting for child survival up

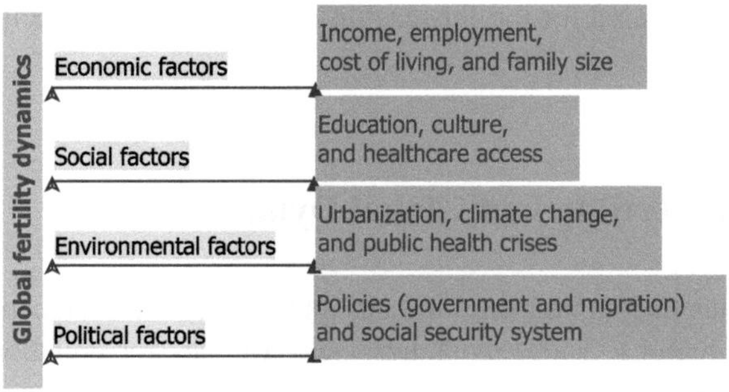

Fig. 1.2 Chart illustrating global fertility dynamics influenced by four main factors: economic, social, environmental, and political [28]. Economic factors include income, employment, cost of living, and family size. Social factors encompass education, culture, and healthcare access. Environmental factors involve urbanization, climate change, and public health crises. Political factors cover government and migration policies, and social security systems

to 15 years, indicates a scenario of population expansion. This parameter, known as TFR, represents the replacement rate [29].

Economic development

Fertility and economic growth share a significant interconnection that shapes the course of societal advancement. Notably, a strong inverse correlation exists between GDP and fertility rates. It is widely acknowledged that reducing family size can augment child development quality and quantity. As economies grow, industrial advancements and technological progress tend to foster enhanced child well-being, leading to a trend of smaller family sizes [30]. However, the "demographic transition" is another pivotal facet of this dynamic. This transition is propelled by factors encompassing improved healthcare, expanded educational opportunities, and the increased participation of women in the workforce [27].

Education and empowerment

Empowerment is considered a means for creating a social environment where vital decisions may be made, and choices can bring social transformation. It strengthens innate ability through acquiring knowledge, power, and experience. The prime factors, such as women's education, working status, involvement in household decision-making, participation in economic decision-making, and freedom of movement, influenced human fertility. In any country, women's empowerment is recognized as a critical factor in reversing the fertility trends. Women with secondary or higher education have a significantly smaller chance of having more births than those with primary education or illiteracy [31].

Family planning and healthcare

These two factors are essential in shaping the TFR and overall population dynamics. Family planning fulfils three vital purposes: averting unintended pregnancies, curtailing the transmission of sexually transmitted diseases, and mitigating infertility rates [32]. Similarly, within the healthcare domain, three pivotal elements come to the forefront: maternal and child health, health education, and medical advancements. Adequate healthcare during pregnancy, childbirth, and early childhood directly reduces child mortality rates, consequently leading to lower fertility rates due to the survival of fewer children. Health education also contributes to preventing infertility through sex education and promoting the adoption of safe contraceptive methods. Furthermore, effective birth spacing, a family planning component, promotes healthier reproductive practices. Extended intervals between births are correlated with diminished fertility rates. Moreover, advancements in medical technology have elevated the success rates of ART, facilitating increased chances of achieving pregnancy [33].

Cultural and religious factors

Faith and religious influence can notably impact the TFR at the individual and national levels. Various cultural elements interplay with fertility, including marriage systems, family structures, religious frameworks, regional subcultures, desired family size norms, and fertility-related practices like astrology and breastfeeding [34]. In some parts of the world, population growth has been accompanied by increased religious devotion. Studies have indicated that strong religiosity correlates with higher TFR values [35].

Urbanization

Urbanization involves the migration of populations from rural regions to urban hubs and can markedly shape human fertility patterns. This phenomenon is frequently linked to alterations in lifestyle, economic prospects, educational and healthcare access, and cultural transformations—factors that collectively influence fertility rates. Urban settings often prompt a preference for smaller family sizes, driven by factors such as increased living expenses, spatial constraints, and evolving social norms. Insight drawn from discrete-time event history analysis has indicated that urban women tend to manifest fertility rates approximately 11% lower than their rural counterparts, although the effects exhibit variability based on parity [36].

Environmental concern

Recent studies have illuminated the link between environmental pollutants and human reproductive challenges, particularly pertaining to infertility. Notably, endocrine-disrupting chemicals, heavy metals, and smoking have emerged as significant factors within the purview of environmental concerns. These chemical pollutants are pervasive in our surroundings, leading to virtually unavoidable human exposure. However, the precise degree to which ecological exposures contribute to infertility remains a subject of uncertainty. Furthermore, occupational exposures and chemical contaminants can adversely affect human fertility and the outcomes of ART. The spectrum of environmental contaminants encompasses various substances, including heavy metals, organic solvents, pesticides, and endocrine-disrupting chemicals [37].

Aging population

The prevailing global demographic trend is the aging of populations, characterized by a transformative evolution in their structural composition over time. This gradual shift has exerted noteworthy and nuanced impacts on social and economic well-being. The interplay between an aging population and fertility is profoundly interconnected. Prolonged lifespans and fertility rates notably below the replacement threshold of 2.1 births per woman have propelled rapid population aging across numerous countries [37]. Recent analysis of transfer accounts data underscores that approximately 48% of the global population resides in countries where the TFR falls below the replacement level. This level of around 2.1 births per woman marks a pivotal tipping point. Furthermore, as persistently low fertility persists, the trajectory of population growth is anticipated to shift towards decline. This decline intensifies the momentum of population aging. As a result, population aging assumes a central role as a "major concern," propelling endeavours to enhance fertility rates [38].

Global migration

Global migration is a complex and multifaceted phenomenon that reflects the aspirations, challenges, and opportunities of individuals seeking better lives and opportunities across borders. It significantly impacts societies, economies, cultures, and global dynamics. The relationship between global migration and fertility is intricate; several factors have influenced it [39]. These factors include cultural norms, access to healthcare, economic conditions in the host country, age at migration, and adaptation to the host country. Hence, migration can have implications for fertility rates in sending and receiving countries, contributing to demographic changes and reshaping future population dynamics [40].

Considering various timeframes, it becomes evident that a multitude of factors significantly impact human fertility. In early life stages, individuals often experience heightened fertility. However, it is important to highlight that many highly developed nations grapple with remarkably low fertility rates, carrying profound implications for their global dynamics. The following discourse delves into prevalent features characterizing fertility challenges, primarily centered around the TFR. A comprehensive examination is conducted to gain a thorough understanding of their significance, encompassing both the top five and low TFR countries. This approach yields valuable insights into the core factors that shape fertility trends.

1.2.1 Proposal 1: Human Fertility and Population Metrics

The TFR is a critical metric that profoundly impacts human population trends. It plays a direct role in determining whether a country's population is growing or declining. When the TFR surpasses the replacement level, it signifies population growth, while a TFR below this threshold indicates a shrinking population. According to rankings provided by "Our World in Data" and the "United Nations Population Fund," the top five countries with notably high TFRs include Niger, Chad, Somalia, the Democratic Republic of Congo (DR Congo), and the Central African Republic. These countries are characterized by several contributing factors that drive their high TFRs, including limited access to contraception, early marriage practices, restricted educational opportunities, elevated maternal mortality rates, constrained healthcare access, reliance on agriculture, challenges in family planning, and gender inequality (see Fig. 1.3a).

Niger stands out with the world's highest fertility rate, averaging around seven children per woman. Its fertility rate is estimated at 6.73 children per woman, leading to a high population growth rate. Niger's population is expected to increase from about 23 million in 2019 to approximately 30 million by 2030. Chad is another country with a relatively high TFR of 5.319, resulting in a current birth rate of 39.913 per 1000 people. The population is projected to grow by 589,234 people, reaching 18,433,996 by the beginning of 2024. In the Democratic Republic of Congo, the estimated TFR is 4.19 in 2023, with a current population of 9,682,157. In the long term,

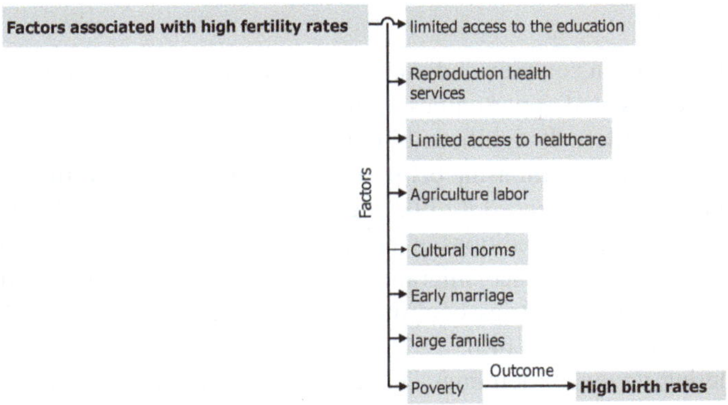

Fig. 1.3 **a** Chart illustrating factors associated with high fertility rates leading to high birth rates. The chart lists factors such as limited access to education, reproductive health services, limited access to healthcare, agricultural labour, cultural norms, early marriage, large families, and poverty. These factors are connected to the outcome of high birth rates. **b** Line chart showing birth rates from 1950 to 2021 for Somalia, Chad, Niger, the Democratic Republic of Congo, the Central African Republic, and the world [41]. The *y*-axis represents births per woman, ranging from 0 to 8. Somalia, Chad, Niger, Democratic Republic of Congo, and the Central African Republic have higher birth rates compared to the global average, which shows a declining trend over time

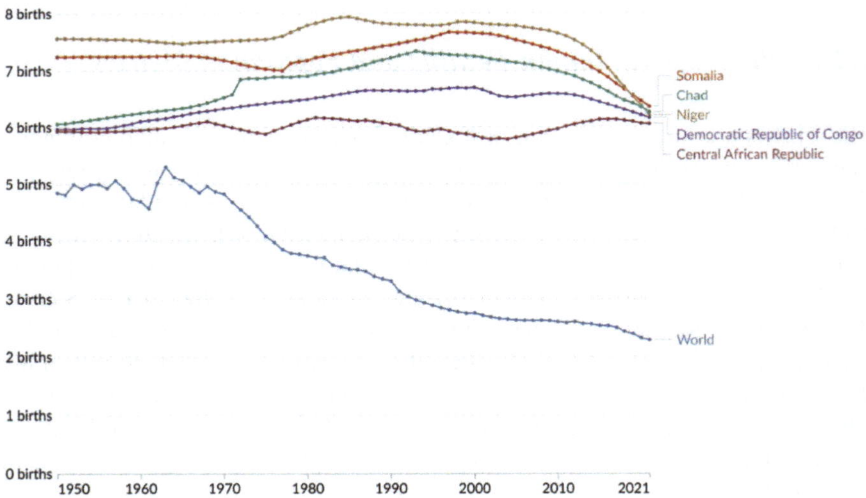

Fig. 1.3 (continued)

the population is expected to stabilize around 98.75 million in 2024. Somalia has an estimated TFR of 5.66, resulting in a birth rate of 40.88 per 1000 people. The current population is approximately 18,143,378, and it is projected to stabilize at around 18.00 million in 2024. The Central African Republic has a TFR of 4.377 and a birth rate of 32.79 per 1000 population. The estimated current population is 102,824,776, projected to stabilize at around 98.75 million. This population represents approximately 1.27% of the world's total population. These African countries demonstrate significantly higher fertility rates compared to many developed nations, leading to substantial population growth. Figure 1.3b offers a visual comparison, illustrating the TFRs of these top 5 countries concerning the global TFR, emphasizing the diversity in demographic patterns across different regions.

In recent years, Taiwan, South Korea, Singapore, Hong Kong, and Macau have all experienced significantly low TFRs, with levels well below the replacement rate of 2.1 children per woman. This decline can be attributed to a complex interplay of social, economic, cultural, and demographic factors. Taiwan, for example, has seen its TFR drop to 1.23 in 2022 from a much higher 5.60 in the early 1900s (see Fig. 1.4a). The country's population, which accounts for about 0.3% of the world's total population, decreased to approximately 23.26 million in 2022. The annual population growth rate has also steadily declined over the years, from 3.90% in 1950 to just 0.13% in recent years. South Korea, often cited as having the world's lowest fertility rate, saw its TFR plummet to 0.8 in 2021, down from 2.1 in 1983. This dramatic change has profoundly impacted the country's annual population growth rate, which reached -0.2% in 2021. South Korea's population represents about 0.64% of the world's total population. Singapore has also experienced a historic low TFR, dropping to 1.05 in 2022 from 2.1 in 1975. The annual population growth rate has fluctuated, with rates of 0.74 in 2020 and 0.65 in 2023. Projections indicate a slight increase in the TFR to 1.06 by 2025. Hong Kong's TFR declined to 0.8 in 2022, marking a significant decrease from 3.2 births per woman in 1973.

Fluctuations in TFR and the annual percentage change in population have been observed. The growth rate was 0.04% in 2023, down from 1.34% in 2020. Projections suggest a TFR of 0.87 by 2030. Lastly, Macau's TFR stands at 1.13, with an annual change in population growth of 1.29%. Forecasts anticipate an increase in both TFR and the growth rate, reaching 1.17 and 1.31, respectively, by 2025. These five developed countries have maintained TFRs below the replacement level for over three decades, typically ranging from 0.9 to 1.3. Factors contributing to these low fertility rates include declining marriage rates, high living costs, easy access to contraception, a lack of work-life support, and other societal and economic influences. Figure 1.4b illustrates the TFR of the countries mentioned above.

To gain a more precise understanding, let's focus on the TFR of the top five developed countries: Norway, Switzerland, Iceland, Hong Kong, and Australia. Norway's TFR stands at 1.6, while Austria has a slightly higher rate at 1.7, though it has seen a gradual decline since 1990, with a more significant drop reported since 2011. Switzerland's TFR, at 1.46, falls below the replacement rate of 2.1. Notably, Switzerland has witnessed a decline in fertility rates since the 1940s, when it stood at four births per woman. In contrast, Hong Kong's TFR is strikingly low at 0.87, representing a substantial departure from the replacement rate. Meanwhile, Iceland's TFR is 1.72, declining from a high of 4.9 births per woman to 2.8 in 1940. These diverse fertility trends underscore the unique demographic challenges and shifts experienced by each of these developed nations. In Fig. 1.5, describe the TFR across the top five developed countries TFR which is compared to the world TFR.

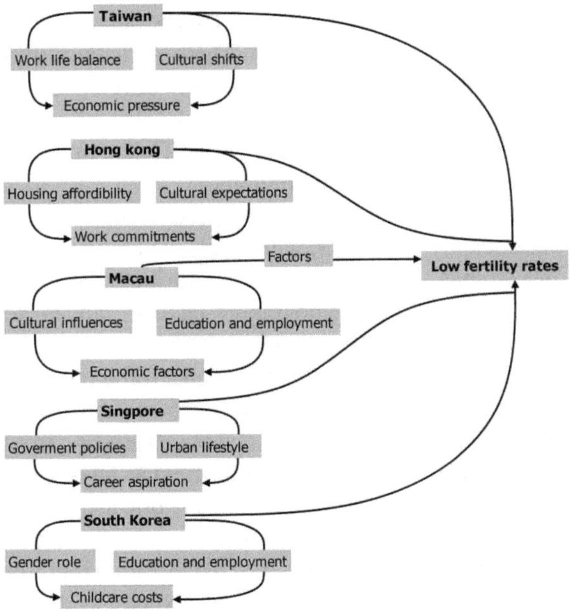

Fig. 1.4 **a** Flow chart illustrating factors contributing to low fertility rates in five regions: Taiwan, Hong Kong, Macau, Singapore, and South Korea. Each region lists specific influences. Taiwan: work-life balance, cultural shifts, economic pressure. Hong Kong: housing affordability, cultural expectations, work commitments. Macau: cultural influences, education and employment, economic factors. Singapore: government policies, urban lifestyle, career aspiration. South Korea: gender role, education and employment, childcare costs. All factors converge towards low fertility rates. **b** Line chart showing the decline in birth rates from 1950 to 2021 for Taiwan, Singapore, South Korea, Hong Kong, and Macao compared to the global average [41]. The y-axis represents the number of births per woman, ranging from 0 to 7, while the x-axis spans the years 1950 to 2021. Each region is represented by a distinct coloured line, with a legend on the right indicating the corresponding colours. The chart highlights a general downward trend in birth rates over time

In addition to the aforementioned countries, several other developed nations, including Denmark, Canada, Sweden, Germany, Spain, and others, have also experienced notably lower TFRs than the replacement rate. In response to this demographic challenge, the concept of a "strategy for reproduction and family life" has been introduced. This strategy aims to tackle the issue of declining fertility rates. It underscores the importance of reproduction in achieving a balanced family life, promoting diversity, enhancing socio-economic equality, and driving progress within communities. To effectively advance this strategy, it is crucial to encourage collaboration among individual governments, the European Economic Community (EEC), the United Nations, and the World Health Organization (WHO). The structure of the strategy is depicted in Fig. 1.6.

Moreover, population growth rate and TFR are closely intertwined demographic metrics that provide profound insights into a society's population dynamics. The population growth rate quantifies how a population's size changes over time,

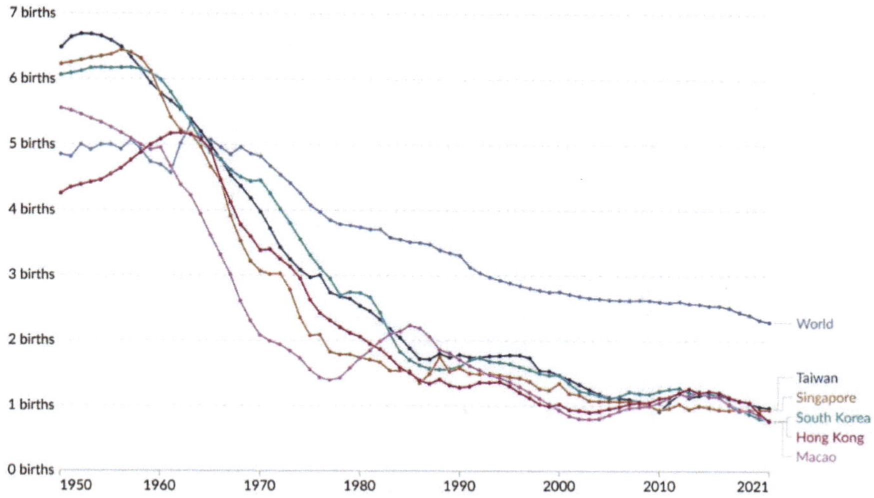

Fig. 1.4 (continued)

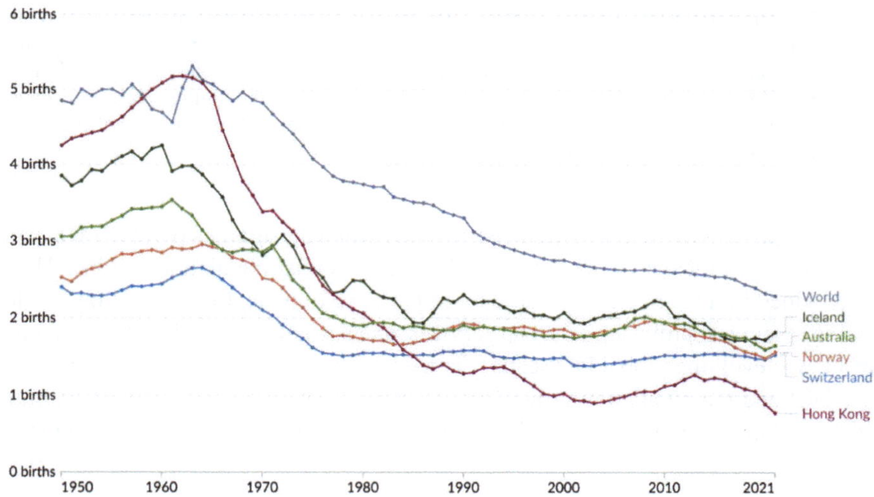

Fig. 1.5 Line chart showing the decline in birth rates from 1950 to 2021 for the world and specific regions: Iceland, Australia, Norway, Switzerland, and Hong Kong [42]. The y-axis represents the number of births per woman, ranging from 0 to 6, while the x-axis shows the years. Each region is represented by a different coloured line, with a general downward trend observed across all regions. The world average starts higher and decreases steadily, while Hong Kong shows the steepest decline

accounting for births, deaths, and net migration, offering a direct measure of demographic shifts within a region. Conversely, TFR reflects the average number of children a woman is expected to have during her reproductive years and acts as a fundamental catalyst for population growth. A TFR exceeding the replacement

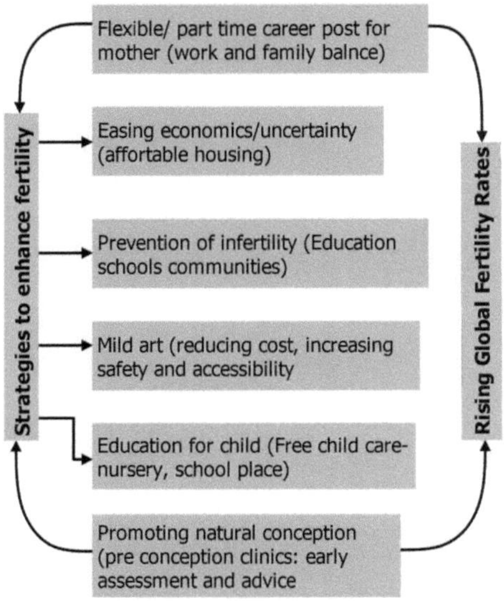

Fig. 1.6 Chart illustrating strategies to enhance fertility and their impact on rising global fertility rates [28]. The chart includes six strategies: "Flexible/part-time career post for mother (work and family balance)," "Easing economics/uncertainty (affordable housing)," "Prevention of infertility (education, schools, communities)," "Mild ART (reducing cost, increasing safety and accessibility)," "Education for child (free childcare, nursery, school place)," and "Promoting natural conception (pre-conception clinics: early assessment and advice)." Arrows connect these strategies to the central theme of enhancing fertility, leading to increased global fertility rates

level of approximately 2.1 children per woman typically signifies population expansion, while a TFR below this threshold hints at potential population decline. These intertwined indicators are of paramount importance to policymakers, aiding in allocating resources, provision of social services, and sustainable development planning in an ever-evolving global landscape. Figure 1.7 illustrates the relationship between the TFR and the population growth rate in various categories, including low, high, and developed countries, by depicting the recent fertility status and demographic trends.

1.2.2 Proposal 2: TFR and GDP

Generally, GDP is a vital gauge for assessing a nation's economic well-being and overall prosperity, offering valuable insights into its economic activities. In parallel, the TFR functions as a statistical measure that provides a comprehensive understanding of fertility patterns within a population, specifically quantifying the average number of children per woman. These two metrics are frequently employed to explore the connection between a country's fertility patterns and its economic standing. While

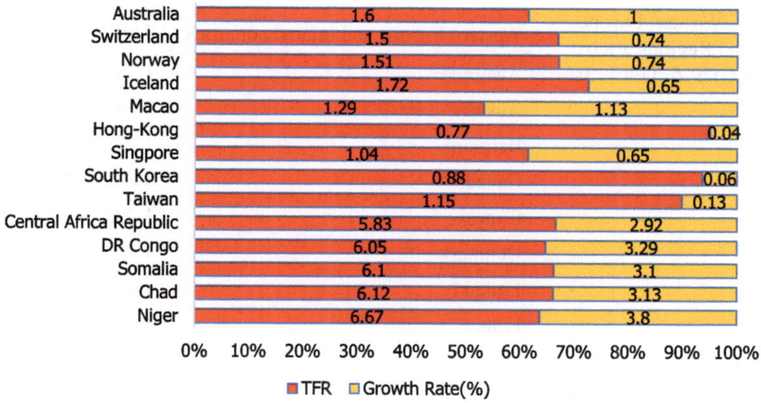

Fig. 1.7 Bar chart comparing Total Fertility Rate (TFR) and Growth Rate (%) across various countries. Countries listed include Australia, Switzerland, Norway, Iceland, Macao, Hong Kong, Singapore, South Korea, Taiwan, the Central African Republic, DR Congo, Somalia, Chad, and Niger. Red bars represent TFR, and yellow bars represent Growth Rate. The chart shows higher TFR and Growth Rates in countries like Niger and Chad, while lower values are observed in countries like Singapore and South Korea. A legend indicates red for TFR and yellow for Growth Rate

they are distinct indicators, a relationship is often observed, albeit with variations among countries and regions. Historically, there has been an inverse correlation between fertility and GDP, with increasing GDP often corresponding to a decrease in the number of children per woman. Higher GDP per capita typically accompanies improved access to education, healthcare, and employment, especially for women. This can lead to delayed childbearing and smaller family sizes as individuals and couples prioritize career advancement and a higher standard of living. Social norms, policies, urbanization, cultural factors, and religious beliefs also influence GDP and TFR. However, it is important to note that these patterns are not universal, and substantial variation exists among countries. Furthermore, relationships can evolve over time as societies adapt to new economic, social, and cultural influences. Therefore, a detailed, case-by-case analysis is essential to comprehend this relationship's intricacies fully.

The TFR exhibits significant diversity among global regions, reflecting the intricate interplay of cultural, social, economic, and demographic factors. To comprehensively analyze this diversity, countries have been categorized into six regions: Western Europe and its affiliated countries, Eastern Europe, Latin America and the Caribbean, Arab States, Sub-Saharan Africa, and Asia. Here, a total of 141 countries have been included within these six regions, with smaller population countries excluded due to their limited impact on regional and global TFR figures and their respective economies. The inclusion criteria are based on the availability of data. The data description is presented in tabular form (see Tables 1.1, 1.2, 1.3, 1.4, 1.5 and 1.6). We all listed the life value of TFR and GDP per capita, collected from the United Nations.

Table 1.1 Western Europe and Related Regions, each country's GDP & TFR [43]

Western Europe and related countries	TFR	GDP (USD)
Australia	1.78	61,224
Austria	1.571	56,506
Belgium	1.77	53,422
Canada	1.48	45,719
Cyprus	1.297	30,379
Denmark	1.77	60,414
Finland	1.41	46,994
France	1.84	39,303
Germany	1.61	42,860
Greece	1.263	234,316
Iceland	1.71	57,452
Ireland	1.78	103,588
Israel	2.93	55,535.87
Italy	1.29	33,232
Luxembourg	1.41	108,952
Malta	1.506	31,338
Netherlands	1.68	61,098.87
New Zealand	1.86	46,936.75
Norway	1.7	81,550.00
Portugal	1.35	22,378
Spain	1.39	28,066
Sweden	1.84	55,260
Switzerland	1.55	89,349
UK	1.75	47,374
USA	1.78	63,935

Case 1, Western Europe & Related Countries

Table 1.1 presents a list of 25 countries categorized into two distinct groups: the first group encompasses nations located to the west of the former Soviet Union, while the second group comprises six states with enduring historical and political affiliations to Western Europe, namely Israel, Iceland, the United States, Canada, Australia, and New Zealand.

The current region boasts an average TFR of 1.599 and a GDP per capita of 61,743.33 USD, highlighting its reputation for advanced and high-income economies. Notably, TFRs consistently fall below the replacement threshold of 2.1 children per woman, indicating a sustained pattern of declining birth rates. This trend is particularly evident in countries such as Greece, Italy, and Cyprus, all struggling with TFRs well below replacement levels. Conversely, Israel maintains a relatively higher TFR, suggesting a degree of resilience in its birth rates. Furthermore,

Table 1.2 Eastern Europe regions, each country's GDP and TFR [44]

Eastern European countries	TFR	GDP (USD)
Bosnia Herzegovina	1.22	6251.1
Hungary	1.54	19,385.78
Poland	1.467	16,805
Slovakia	1.552	23,457.54
Czech Republic	1.682	31,368.43
Rumania	1.647	12,623
Croatia	1.407	20,537.08
Ukraine	1.2	2074
Latvia	1.74	17,168
Bulgaria	1.612	9673.00
Slovenia	1.638	32,214
Estonia	1.635	20,995
Serbia	1.421	7545
Lithuania	1.701	18,366.94
Belarus	1.736	7944.77
Armenia	1.758	5290
Montenegro	1.742	8069
Albania	1.545	7058.82
Georgia	2.015	7600.35
Turkey	1.994	14,355

there is a noteworthy variation among nations in terms of economic prosperity, with the majority enjoying financial stability. Countries like Switzerland, Luxembourg, Greece, and Norway, which are perennial leaders in terms of GDP per capita on a global scale, exemplify this economic trend. In this context, these countries have achieved low TFRs of 1.55, 1.41, 1.26, and 1.7, respectively.

Case 2, Eastern Europe

Table 1.2 includes data for a total of 20 countries, including those in Eastern Europe with historical ties to the Soviet Union, as well as Albania, Turkey, and Georgia. The data includes information on TFR and GDP for these countries.

The current region exhibits an average GDP of 14,689.94 USD and a TFR of 1.67. In comparison to Western European nations, this region has a notably lower GDP. Conversely, the TFR in this region falls below the replacement level, suggesting a trend of declining fertility. Notably, the TFR was relatively high in earlier years, but a significant decline occurred after 2015 [45]. For instance, Ukraine and Bosnia Herzegovina have the lowest TFR among all the countries in the region, while Georgia and Turkey have achieved higher TFRs in 2023. However, a few countries in the region have faced more modest GDP per capita figures. These fluctuations in both

Table 1.3 Latin American and the Caribbean regions, each country's GDP and TFR [46]

Latin America and the Caribbean	TFR	GDP (USD)
Brazil	1.668	9034
Trinidad and Tobago	1.672	14,915
Chile	1.598	17,827.41
Costa Rica	1.682	13,935
Columbia	1.727	6995
Uruguay	1.924	21,677.29
Jamaica	1.915	5343
El Salvador	1.957	4396.00
Mexico	2.027	9980
Nicaragua	2.279	2162
Argentina	2.199	13,709.49
Venezuela	2.184	3640.81
Peru	2.162	6725
Dominican Republic	2.235	9064
Ecuador	2.322	5730
Paraguay	2.329	6379
Guyana	2.368	21,859
Panama	2.366	17,350.08
Belize	2.194	6472
Bolivia	2.577	3800.28
Honduras	2.321	3278.01
Haiti	2.745	1240
Guatemala	2.67	5358.21

GDP and TFR are attributed to factors such as political instability, corruption, and economic vulnerabilities.

Case 3, Latin America & The Caribbean

Table 1.3 presents data for a total of 23 countries, which includes all the countries in the Americas located south of the United States. Additionally, four Caribbean countries, namely Trinidad & Tobago, Jamaica, the Dominican Republic, and Haiti, are also included. The data in the table comprises information on GDP and TFR for these countries. The average GDP per capita for this region is 9385 USD, and the average TFR stands at 2.20. Notably, this region reflects an upward trend in fertility rates, with TFR surpassing the replacement level. The countries with the highest TFRs in this region are Bolivia, Haiti, and Guatemala, with GDP per capita ranging from approximately 3000 to 5000 USD. In contrast, the countries with the lowest TFRs in this region are Trinidad & Tobago, Chile, Costa Rica, and Brazil, where TFR values are under 1.6. Interestingly, these countries also have relatively higher GDP

Table 1.4 Arab States regions each country's GDP & TFR [47]

Arab states	TFR	GDP (USD)
Lebanon	2.018	5375
United Arab Emirates	1.354	47,088
Qatar	1.778	66,334
Kuwait	2.031	33,646.14
Bahrain	1.891	25,127
Tunisia	2.096	3960
Libya	2.115	9677.00
Morocco	2.296	3401
Saudi Arabia	2.175	29,922.09
Algeria	2.789	4128
Egypt	3.131	4261
Jordon	2.575	5048.46
Palestinian Terr.	3.2	3157.00
Yemen	3.427	573.19
Iraq	3.446	6180.52
Comoros	3.85	1409
Sudan	4.154	2170
Mauretania	4.321	1686

per capita compared to the nations with higher TFRs. These variations contribute to reshaping the global trends in TFR.

Case 4, Arab States

Table 1.4 presents data for a total of 18 countries situated in Northwestern, Northern, and Northeastern Africa, as well as Western Asia. This includes Iraq and countries in the Arabian Peninsula, though it does not extend further east. The table provides information on TFR and GDP per capita for these countries.

The average GDP in this region stands at 15,019.33 USD, while the average TFR is 2.75. Within this region, the highest TFRs are observed in Sudan and Mauretania, while the United Arab Emirates has the lowest TFR. When it comes to GDP per capita, the highest figure is achieved by the United Arab Emirates, whereas Yemen reports the lowest GDP per capita. Furthermore, some countries in the region, such as Egypt, the Palestinian Territories, and Comoros, demonstrate favourable TFRs. It is important to note that the Arab States in this region are generally experiencing an upward trend in fertility rates.

Case 5, Sub-Saharan Africa

Table 1.5 presents data for 31 countries located south of the Sahara Desert, including Comoros, Sudan, and Mauritania within the Arab States category. This region had the highest average TFR among all regions, approximately 4.1. Similarly, the region

Table 1.5 Sub-Saharan Africa regions, each country's GDP and TFR [48]

Sub-Saharan Africa	TFR	GDP (USD)
Namibia	3.171	5100.23
South Africa	2.309	6043.00
Botswana	2.69	6910
Swaziland	2.839	4159
Zimbabwe	3.32	1376
Kenya	3.259	2269.02
Ghana	3.647	2071
Rwanda	3.731	1014.00
Madagascar	3.854	472.92
Togo	4.06	947.58
Liberia	4.035	805.37
Cierra Leone	3.856	670.00
Congo Brazzaville	4.194	571.09
Mali	5.461	567.50
Cameroon	4.295	1508
Senegal	4.342	1606
Central African Republic	4.377	369.82
Guinea	4.377	994.44
Ivory Coast	2.97	2581
Gambia	4.904	719.73
Benin	4.543	1332
Tanzania	4.629	1112
Mozambique	4.542	609.77
Burkina Faso	4.835	767.49
Nigeria	5.076	2523
Uganda	4.435	1105.36
Burundi	5.045	249.22
Chad	5.319	610.38
Mali	5.461	786.12
Congo Kinshasa	4.194	571.09
Niger	6.73	578.19

had the lowest average GDP per capita, which stood at 1699.27 USD. Notably, within these 31 nations, specific countries such as South Africa and the Ivory Coast stand out due to their comparatively low TFRs. This contrasts with countries like Chad, Niger, Burundi, Nigeria, the Democratic Republic of Congo, and Mali, which exhibit higher TFR rates.

Table 1.6 Asia regions, each country's GDP and TFR [49]

Asia	TFR	GDP (USD)
Hong Kong	1.413	44,931
Singapore	1.244	91,100.37
South Korea	1.075	34,149.00
Japan	1.367	4409.74
Thailand	1.461	8181.93
Iran	2.091	4251.67
Vietnam	2.019	3875
Azerbaijan	1.993	6938.800
Malaysia	1.924	11,884
Bangladesh	1.93	1883
Myanmar	2.073	1180.48
Nepal	1.799	1399.01
Uzbekistan	2.309	3630
India	2.0	2221
Indonesia	2.22	4277
Cambodia	2.394	1583
Kazakhstan	2.622	11,822
Mongolia	2.731	4354
Laos	2.3	2729
Philippines	2.454	3768
Kyrgyzstan	2.9	1266
Tajikistan	3.404	1277.91
Pakistan	3.238	1543
Afghanistan	3.851	410.03

Regarding GDP figures, countries such as Niger, Burundi, and the Democratic Republic of Congo (Congo Kinshasa) have the lowest values. In contrast, Namibia, South Africa, and Botswana report relatively higher GDP figures.

Case 6, Asia

Table 1.6 provides data for 24 countries located in Central, Eastern, and Southern Asia. This region is exceptionally diverse, comprising countries that share certain cultural and political characteristics, albeit with significant variations. The table includes GDP per capita figures and TFR values for these countries.

The region exhibits an average TFR of 2.20 and an approximate GDP per capita of 10,074.62 USD. It is common to observe variations in TFR within regions. For instance, South Korea has the lowest TFR at 1.075, while Afghanistan has the highest TFR among all countries in the region. This stark contrast in TFR is mirrored in the economic conditions, with South Korea enjoying a robust economy, whereas

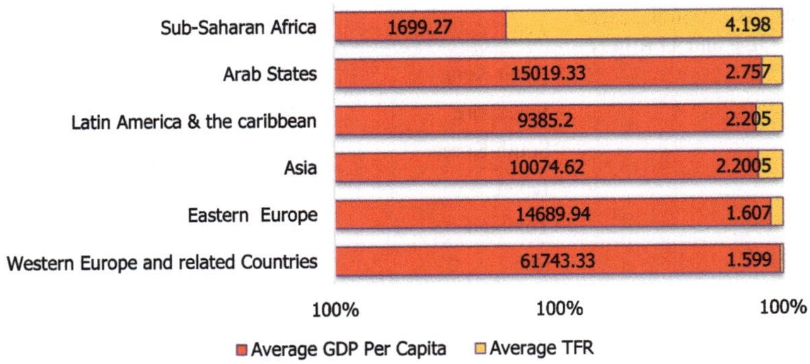

Fig. 1.8 Bar chart comparing average GDP per capita and average Total Fertility Rate (TFR) across different regions. Regions include Sub-Saharan Africa, Arab States, Latin America and the Caribbean, Asia, Eastern Europe, Western Europe and related countries. Each region has two bars: one for GDP per capita in red and one for TFR in yellow. Sub-Saharan Africa shows the lowest GDP and highest TFR, while Western Europe shows the highest GDP and lowest TFR. The chart highlights economic and demographic differences between regions

Afghanistan faces economic challenges. Similarly, Singapore stands out with a higher GDP and a lower TFR (1.22). However, it is worth noting that nine countries in the region have TFRs lower than the replacement level, while 11 are just slightly above the replacement value. Consequently, the overall TFR picture for Asian countries indicates an upward trend in fertility rates.

The data reveals an intriguing pattern where regions with lower TFRs exhibit higher GDP per capita values than areas with higher TFRs. Figure 1.8 comprehensively overviews the relationship between GDP and TFR among 141 countries. Therefore, a robust correlation between GDP and TFR indicates that economic growth significantly influences a country's TFR.

1.2.3 Proposal 3: TFR and HDI

HDI and TFR are pivotal indicators for evaluating a country's population well-being and development. Understanding the interplay between HDI and TFR is paramount, as it offers valuable insights into a nation's developmental status. This assessment is underpinned by four core factors: socio-economic development, the impact of education, healthcare and life expectancy, and living standards. Therefore, the integration of these four elements is crucial when evaluating TFR. HDI scores are condensed into a single number ranging from 0 to 1.0, and they are categorized into four tiers: very high (0.8–1), high (0.7–0.79), medium (0.55–0.70), and low (below 0.55). Most developed countries typically have an HDI score of 0.8 or higher, reflecting a high standard of living, robust healthcare services, and strong educational systems.

Conversely, the lowest HDI score of 0.55 or below signifies a poor standard of living, limited access to healthcare services, and inadequate education. In this context, we delve into the correlation between HDI and TFR by scrutinizing the top 10 countries with the highest HDI scores alongside the bottom 10 countries with the lowest HDI scores. This analysis provides valuable insights into the interconnection between these critical development indicators, helping us understand the relationship between well-being and fertility rates.

Case 1, Top 10 countries with the highest HDI

According to the 2021 World Population Prospects, several countries are noteworthy for their high HDI scores. The top 10 HDI countries in this ranking are Switzerland, Norway, Iceland, Hong Kong, Australia, Denmark, Sweden, Ireland, Germany, and the Netherlands. These nations excel in multiple dimensions, offering a superior standard of living, robust healthcare services, excellent access to education, high literacy rates, and substantial sources of income and social connections. As a result, these countries provide a fulfilling life for their residents, reflecting an elevated quality of life and robust economic conditions. Remarkably, research in this field consistently indicates that countries with higher HDI scores tend to exhibit lower TFR [50]. Figure 1.9 visually depicts the precise relationship between TFR and HDI, offering a clear graphical representation that facilitates a deeper understanding of the significant impact of HDI on human fertility. According to Our World in Data, historical changes have been noted since the 1990s when the HDI scores ranged between 0.3 and 0.5, and the TFR was at 2.4, which was above the replacement level. In contrast, the current scenario shows that despite high HDI scores, there has been a noticeable impact on TFR, which has dropped below the replacement level. However, on a global scale, the TFR stands at 2.3, indicating that the declining fertility rate is more prominent in countries with the highest HDI scores.

Case 2, Top 10 countries with the lowest HDI

The 2021 version of the HDI report underscores those countries with HDI scores below 0.5 indicate a low standard of living for their citizens. The ten countries with the lowest HDI scores are South Sudan, Chad, Niger, the Central African Republic, Burundi, Mali, Mozambique, Burkina Faso, Yemen, and Guinea. It is worth noting that most of these countries are situated in the Sub-Saharan Africa region. As widely recognized, Chad, Niger, the Central African Republic, and Mali have some of the highest TFR globally, despite their remarkably low HDI values. A striking example is South Sudan, with a TFR of 4.5, while its HDI score stands at a notably low 0.385, garnering attention worldwide. Figure 1.10 provides a visual representation of the lowest HDI scores among these ten countries and their corresponding TFRs, highlighting the challenges they face in terms of both development and fertility rates.

According to the figure, the Human Development Index scores follow a nearly linear pattern across all the presented countries, while the Total Fertility Rate varies considerably. The TFR typically ranges from 3.8 to 6.8, with Niger recording the highest value and Yemen one of the lowest at 3.8. Notably, despite having the lowest HDI value among these countries, South Sudan maintains a TFR of 4.5. In the early

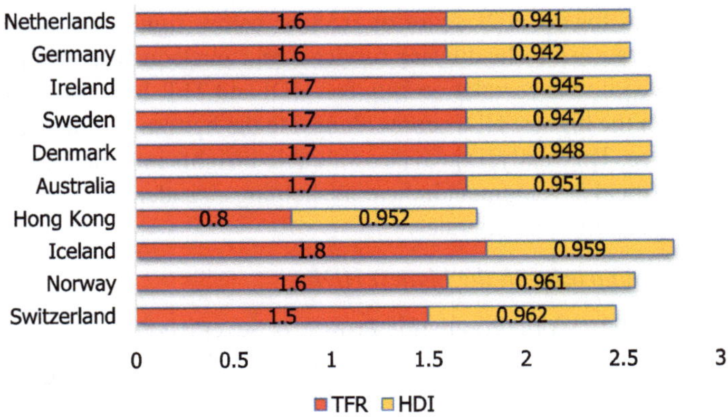

Fig. 1.9 Horizontal bar chart comparing the TFR (red) and HDI (yellow) for various countries. Countries listed include the Netherlands, Germany, Finland, Sweden, Denmark, Australia, Hong Kong, Iceland, Norway, and Switzerland [51]. Each bar is divided into two segments representing the TFR and HDI values, with numerical values labelled on the bars. The chart highlights differences in these indices across the countries

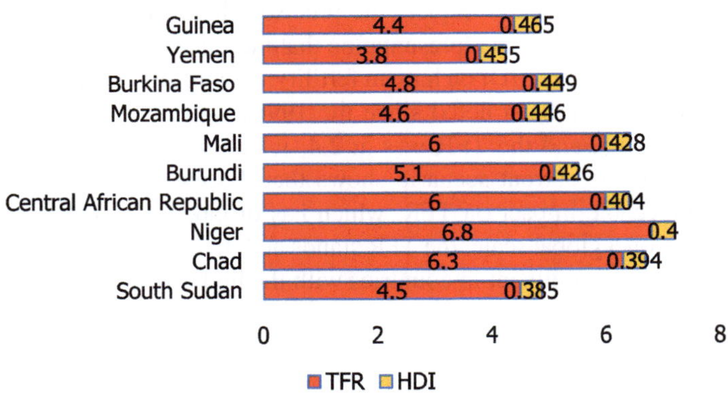

Fig. 1.10 Bar chart comparing Total Fertility Rate (TFR) and Human Development Index (HDI) for various countries [51]. Countries listed include Guinea, Yemen, Burkina Faso, Mozambique, Mali, Burundi, the Central African Republic, Niger, Chad, and South Sudan. TFR values are represented in red bars, while HDI values are shown in yellow bars. The chart highlights differences in TFR and HDI across these countries, with TFR values generally higher than HDI values. A legend at the bottom indicates the colour coding for TFR and HDI

1900s, the HDI was predominantly in the range of 0.02 to 0.1, and concurrently, the TFR consistently exceeded 7. This historical context starkly contrasts with contemporary figures, emphasizing significantly lower HDI levels and notably higher fertility rates. It serves as a compelling reminder of how development indicators have evolved. Furthermore, the visual representation in Fig. 1.10 strongly suggests a clear association between higher fertility rates and lower HDI scores. This underscores the concept that as HDI declines, there is a tendency toward higher fertility rates in these regions.

1.2.4 Proposal 4: TFR and Social Factors

Social factors play a pivotal role in driving changes in population dynamics, especially when it comes to their influence on fertility rates. Fertility rates are a cornerstone of population trends, and various social determinants can sway individuals and couples in their decisions to have more or fewer children. Extensive surveys have been conducted to pinpoint the impact of social factors on fertility rates. A notable global trend has emerged in recent years, particularly during the last decade of the twentieth century: a decline in TFR across many countries. To illustrate, in the early 1950s, the global TFR stood at 5, decreasing to 4.5 by the early 1970s and dropping below three by 1990 [52]. This decline is particularly prominent in developing countries, with Asia, North Africa, and Latin America experiencing the most rapid reductions in TFR, owing to their stable socio-economic development. Remarkably, in 2019, the Middle East and North Africa (MENA) region witnessed a substantial decrease in fertility rates [53]. Countries like Lebanon, Egypt, the Islamic Republic of Iran, and Turkey have achieved TFRs below the replacement level. A blend of social factors, including diverse cultures, religious beliefs, family structures, and education levels, influences these shifts in TFR. These social conditions collectively contribute to shaping the overall TFR landscape globally [54].

Condition 1, Religiosity

The world's primary religions are commonly classified into two main categories: Abrahamic and Indian religions. Among the Abrahamic faiths, three major groups are recognized, including Christianity, Islam, and Judaism, while within the Indian religious sphere, Hinduism, Buddhism, and Sikhism are the predominant traditions. Notably, Christianity is the most prominent global religion, boasting a following of two billion adherents, with Islam ranking as the second most widely practiced religion, with 1.8 billion followers. Conversely, Hinduism is estimated to have 1.1 billion adherents, and Buddhism counts approximately 500 million followers. Thus, these four religions are practiced extensively worldwide, each characterized by its distinct set of beliefs, rituals, and traditions. Importantly, these four major religions can significantly influence global population strategies, with the TFR playing a pivotal role in shaping demographic trends. Furthermore, it is well-documented that varying degrees of religiosity can impact fertility patterns, underscoring the role of faith in this context.

A recent study conducted across 141 European countries revealed a notable correlation between religiosity and fertility rates, indicating that higher religiosity correlates with higher fertility [55]. According to global population growth projections, Islam exhibits rapid growth with a TFR of 3.1, while Hindus report a TFR of 2.4. In comparison, Christians and Buddhists have TFRs of 2.7 and 1.6, respectively. When these rates are compared with the global TFR of 2.5, Muslims have the highest fertility, followed by Christians, with Hindu fertility almost aligning with the worldwide average. Certain religions, such as folk traditions, unaffiliated groups, and Buddhists, have TFRs below the replacement level (2.1), indicating declining populations. In contrast, Jewish fertility rates are above replacement levels, highlighting the diverse fertility patterns across religious groups.

As per country-level projections, Sub-Saharan Africa is anticipated to undergo rapid population growth, particularly among Christians, who comprise 62% of the population and are expected to double. Additionally, Muslims constitute approximately 31.4% of the total population, while 3.2% practice traditional African religions, and 3% adhere to unaffiliated beliefs. In contrast, Taiwan, located in Asia, exhibits the lowest TFR. Predominantly influenced by Buddhism and Taoism, most of Taiwan's population follows these traditions, with only 4.5% identifying as Christian and 0.3% as Muslims. These demographic trends highlight the significant role of diverse religious beliefs in shaping fertility patterns, with Africa demonstrating the highest TFR and Taiwan representing the lowest, reflecting the impact of various faiths on population growth [55, 56].

Condition 2, Family system

Family systems encompass the intricate web of norms, values, and practices governing familial relationships within distinct cultural contexts. These systems exhibit considerable diversity across societies, shaped by factors like household composition and family roles. They are closely intertwined with TFR, making this relationship complex and multifaceted. A wealth of literature explores the interplay between family structures and TFR, emphasizing the need to understand these dynamics for effective population planning. In 1990, a study in Chennai revealed that joint families tended to have higher fertility rates, while nuclear families exhibited the lowest fertility rates [57].

Similarly, in 2018, a European study investigated the influence of family systems on fertility and found that the effects varied based on individuals' intentions to start or expand their families [58]. For those without children, reduced proximity to relatives was linked to less favourable attitudes toward parenthood, whereas individuals already parenting benefited from the presence of close family members. India's family system differs significantly from Western countries. Weak kin ties, high cohabitation rates, and smaller households are prevalent in Northwestern Europe. At the same time, Southern European families maintain strong kin connections, have lower cohabitation rates, and have more complex household structures on average. Eastern Europe shares similarities with Southern Europe but stands out with early marriages and high divorce rates. There has been a notable transition from joint to nuclear family structures in India, contributing to reduced TFR. Smaller family units prioritize better education and improved quality of life, and this transformation underscores the significant influence of family systems on fertility.

Condition 3, Marriage and education

The increase in education levels is thought to be a contributing factor to the declining fertility rates in many countries. Longer and more extensive education empowers women, leading to later marriages, delayed childbearing, and smaller family sizes [59]. The timing of marriage plays a crucial role, as it has historically been closely associated with age, serving as a strong indicator of women's fertility patterns. In Uttar Pradesh, a study was conducted to explore the relationship between the average age at marriage, education, and fertility. Approximately 1000 families participated in the survey, covering a range of ages from 15 to 50 years. The study's results revealed that higher education and later marriage were linked to a reduction in fertility rates [60]. In Saudi Arabia, a case study was conducted among women at King Saud University, revealing a solid connection between fertility and improved education [61]. This extensive study involved 11,390 participants and considered various factors, including background information, marital history, birth history, and desired versus actual family sizes. Theoretically, pursuing education is often preceded by lifestyle changes, including livelihood improvements. These improved livelihood prospects place greater importance on education, which, in turn, increases the costs associated with raising children. Consequently, this can lead to delays in achieving various family-related milestones, such as marriage, childbirth, and home purchases. Such delays significantly impact the fertility of communities, societies, and states. Another case study conducted in Western Europe found that an increasing number of women pursuing professions and careers dampens fertility rates. However, it is worth noting that recent trends indicate a slight reversal in declining fertility rates due to an increase in marriage resulting from higher education and employment opportunities. Legislative efforts to prohibit early marriages have also contributed to this trend [62]. The age at which individuals choose to marry, and their subsequent marital experiences, can profoundly impact their personal well-being and exert far-reaching effects on broader social dynamics. Research has demonstrated that the quality of the marriage relationship is a significant predictor of infertility, leading to marital problems and conflicts with severe implications for mental health [63]. Delayed marriages can disrupt fertility patterns and create stressful conditions. Conversely, early marriages are still prevalent in certain states like Bihar and Uttar Pradesh in India. Adolescent girls who enter early marriages are vulnerable to poor reproductive health outcomes. These young married girls often find themselves in gender-inequitable contexts, contending with pressures related to fertility from their in-laws. Bihar and Uttar Pradesh, characterized by large populations, have witnessed a noticeable decline in contraceptive use over the past decade. There is growing evidence highlighting the influence of social norms, which may limit or entirely deprive adolescent girls of control over their reproductive health, including access to family planning services [64]. Furthermore, it is evident that education and marriage are intricately linked with fertility, and this connection is multifaceted and complex.

1.3 Conclusion and Future Awareness

In shaping future fertility trends and their societal impact, it is imperative to prioritize extensive educational and awareness initiatives concerning reproductive health and family planning. These efforts should be underscored by a strong emphasis on the significance of gender equality and women's empowerment in influencing decisions related to fertility. Ensuring widespread access to a diverse array of family planning methods and providing essential support for individuals grappling with infertility is of paramount importance. Additionally, establishing resilient healthcare systems capable of delivering comprehensive reproductive health services, collecting demographic data, and offering mental health support is crucial. Furthermore, it is vital to address the influence of social norms and values on fertility choices and encourage discussions on the sustainability of global population growth. Collaboration in research and innovation, policy adaptation, cultural sensitivity, and international cooperation should be pivotal elements in steering future fertility trends.

References

1. Roser, M. (2014). The global decline of the fertility rate. *Our world in Data.*
2. Becker, G. (2000). *The elusive embryo: How women and men approach new reproductive technologies.* University of California Press.
3. McQueston, K., Silverman, R., & Glassman, A. (2012). Adolescent fertility in low-and middle-income countries: Effects and solutions. *Center for Global Development Working Paper, 295.*
4. Mascarenhas, M. N., Flaxman, S. R., Boerma, T., Vanderpoel, S., & Stevens, G. A. (2012). National, regional, and global trends in infertility prevalence since 1990: A systematic analysis of 277 health surveys. *PLoS Medicine, 9*(12), Article e1001356.
5. Leke, R. J., Oduma, J. A., Bassol-Mayagoitia, S., Bacha, A. M., & Grigor, K. M. (1993). Regional and geographical variations in infertility: Effects of environmental, cultural, and socioeconomic factors. *Environmental Health Perspectives, 101*(suppl 2), 73–80.
6. Inhorn, M. C., & Patrizio, P. (2015). Infertility around the globe: New thinking on gender, reproductive technologies and global movements in the 21st century. *Human Reproduction Update, 21*(4), 411–426.
7. Burns, L. H., & Covington, S. N. (2006). Psychology of infertility. In *Infertility counseling: A comprehensive handbook for clinicians* (pp. 1–19).
8. Aneshensel, C. S., & Sucoff, C. A. (1996). The neighborhood context of adolescent mental health. *Journal of Health and Social Behavior*, 293–310.
9. Becker, G. (2022). *Healing the infertile family: Strengthening your relationship in the search for parenthood.* University of California Press.
10. Hwang, T. J., Rabheru, K., Peisah, C., Reichman, W., & Ikeda, M. (2020). Loneliness and social isolation during the COVID-19 pandemic. *International Psychogeriatrics, 32*(10), 1217–1220.
11. Umberson, D., & Karas Montez, J. (2010). Social relationships and health: A flashpoint for health policy. *Journal of Health and Social Behavior, 51*(1_suppl), S54–S66.
12. Iordăchescu, D. A., Golu, F. T., Paica, C. I., Gorbănescu, A., Panaitescu, A. M., Gică, C., Peltecu, G., & Gică, N., (2021, November). The Relationship between the Infertility Specialist and the Patient during the COVID-19 Pandemic. *Healthcare, 9,* (12), 1649.
13. Graham, M. E., Jelin, A., Hoon, A. H., Jr., Wilms Floet, A. M., Levey, E., & Graham, E. M. (2023). Assisted reproductive technology: Short-and long-term outcomes. *Developmental Medicine & Child Neurology, 65*(1), 38–49.

14. Tamir, S. (2023). Artificial intelligence in human reproduction: Charting the ethical debate over AI in IVF. *AI and Ethics, 3*(3), 947–961.
15. Opara, H. C., Iheanacho, P. N., Nebo, B., Ingwu, J. A., Anetekhai, C. J., & Anarado, A. N. (2022). Factors affecting adherence to anti-retroviral therapy among women attending HIV clinic of a tertiary health institution in SouthEastern, Nigeria. *African Health Sciences, 22*(1), 456–464.
16. Emokpae, M. A., & Brown, S. I. (2021). Effects of lifestyle factors on fertility: Practical recommendations for modification. *Reproduction and Fertility, 2*(1), R13–R26.
17. Kundu, S., Ali, B., & Dhillon, P. (2023). Surging trends of infertility and its behavioural determinants in India. *PLoS ONE, 18*(7), Article e0289096.
18. Sharma, R., Biedenharn, K. R., Fedor, J. M., & Agarwal, A. (2013). Lifestyle factors and reproductive health: Taking control of your fertility. *Reproductive Biology and Endocrinology, 11*, 1–15.
19. Petrova, D., Catena, A., Rodríguez-Barranco, M., Redondo-Sánchez, D., Bayo-Lozano, E., Garcia-Retamero, R., Jiménez-Moleón, J. J., & Sánchez, M. J. (2021). Physical comorbidities and depression in recent and long-term adult cancer survivors: NHANES 2007–2018. *Cancers, 13*(13), 3368.
20. Biondi, B., Kahaly, G. J., & Robertson, R. P. (2019). Thyroid dysfunction and diabetes mellitus: Two closely associated disorders. *Endocrine Reviews, 40*(3), 789–824.
21. Lorzadeh, N., Kazemirad, N., & Kazemirad, Y. (2020). Human immunodeficiency: Extragonadal comorbidities of infertility in women. *Immunity, Inflammation and Disease, 8*(3), 447–457.
22. Dinsdale, N. L., & Crespi, B. J. (2021). Endometriosis and polycystic ovary syndrome are diametric disorders. *Evolutionary Applications, 14*(7), 1693–1715.
23. Eisenberg, M. L., Sundaram, R., Maisog, J., & Buck Louis, G. M. (2016). Diabetes, medical comorbidities and couple fecundity. *Human Reproduction, 31*(10), 2369–2376.
24. Slavich, G. M. (2022). Social Safety Theory: Understanding social stress, disease risk, resilience, and behavior during the COVID-19 pandemic and beyond. *Current Opinion in Psychology, 45*, Article 101299.
25. Hoek, A., Wang, Z., van Oers, A. M., Groen, H., & Cantineau, A. E. (2022). Effects of preconception weight loss after lifestyle intervention on fertility outcomes and pregnancy complications. *Fertility and Sterility, 118*(3), 456–462.
26. https://data.worldbank.org/indicator/SP.DYN.TFRT.IN. Last accessed November, 5.
27. Kruk, M. E., Gage, A. D., Arsenault, C., Jordan, K., Leslie, H. H., Roder-DeWan, S., Adeyi, O., Barker, P., Daelmans, B., Doubova, S. V., English, M., García-Elorrio, E., Guanais, F., Gureje, O., Hirschhorn, L. R., Jiang, L., Kelley, E., Lemango, E. T., Liljestrand, J., …, Pate, M. (2018). High-quality health systems in the Sustainable Development Goals era: Time for a revolution. *The Lancet Global Health, 6*(11), e1196–e1252.
28. Bongaarts, J. (2009). Human population growth and the demographic transition. *Philosophical Transactions of the Royal Society B: Biological Sciences, 364*(1532), 2985–2990.
29. O'sullivan, J. N. (2023). Demographic delusions: World population growth is exceeding most projections and jeopardising scenarios for sustainable futures. *World, 4*(3), 545–568.
30. Zhang, X., Guan, Q., Yu, Q., Xiao, W., Chen, Z., Dong, C., Deng, S., Zhuang, Y., & Xia, Y. (2022). Estimating the effects of policies on infertility prevalence worldwide. *BMC Public Health, 22*(1), 1378.
31. Saurabh, S., Sarkar, S., & Pandey, D. K. (2013). Female literacy rate is a better predictor of birth rate and infant mortality rate in India. *Journal of Family Medicine and Primary Care, 2*(4), 349–353.
32. Tsui, A. O., McDonald-Mosley, R., & Burke, A. E. (2010). Family planning and the burden of unintended pregnancies. *Epidemiologic Reviews, 32*(1), 152–174.
33. Fortin, C., & Abele, S. (2015). Increased length of awareness of assisted reproductive technologies fosters positive attitudes and acceptance among women. *International Journal of Fertility & Sterility, 9*(4), 452.

34. Nibhon, D., & Noppavan, C. (1981). Interrelationship of culture and fertility: A review of Thai experience. *Journal of Thai Association for Voluntary Sterilization*, 5–18.
35. Bora, J. K., Saikia, N., Kebede, E. B., & Lutz, W. (2023). Revisiting the causes of fertility decline in Bangladesh: The relative importance of female education and family planning programs. *Asian Population Studies, 19*(1), 81–104.
36. Hashimoto, H., & Naito, T. (2024). Regional differences in childcare environment, urbanization, and fertility decline. *Letters in Spatial and Resource Sciences, 17*(1), 8.
37. Kumar, N., & Singh, A. K. (2022). Impact of environmental factors on human semen quality and male fertility: A narrative review. *Environmental Sciences Europe, 34*, 1–13.
38. Kamwengo, J. (2022). *An exploration into increasing teenage pregnancy in government secondary schools in Lukulu district of western province* [Doctoral dissertation, The University of Zambia].
39. Aitken, R. J. (2022). *The infertility trap: Why life choices impact your fertility and why we must act now*. Cambridge University Press.
40. Miao, R. (2023). Aging Alleviation Through Increasing Fertility and Migration. *Lecture Notes in Education Psychology and Public Media, 13*, 14–19.
41. https://worldpopulationreview.com/country-rankings/total-fertility-rate
42. https://data.worldbank.org/indicator/SP.DYN.TFRT.IN
43. https://ourworldindata.org/grapher/gdp-world-regions-stacked-area
44. https://data.worldbank.org/region/europe-and-central-asia?view=chart
45. https://www.un.org/development/desa/pd/sites/www.un.org.development.desa.pd/files/files/documents/2020/Feb/un_2015_worldfertilityreport_highlights.pdf
46. https://data.worldbank.org/region/latin-america-and-caribbean?view=chart
47. https://data.worldbank.org/indicator/NY.GDP.PCAP.CD?page=4&locations=1A
48. https://data.worldbank.org/region/sub-saharan-africa?view=chart
49. https://data.worldbank.org/region/east-asia-and-pacific?view=chart
50. Furuoka, F. (2009). Looking for a J-shaped development-fertility relationship: Do advances in development really reverse fertility declines. *Economics bulletin, 29*(4), 3067–3074.
51. https://worldpopulationreview.com/country-rankings/hdi-by-country
52. Pourreza, A., Sadeghi, A., Amini-Rarani, M., Khodayari-Zarnaq, R., & Jafari, H. (2021). Contributing factors to the total fertility rate declining trend in the Middle East and North Africa: A systemic review. *Journal of Health, Population and Nutrition, 40*, 1–7.
53. Drioui, C., El Bidaoui, B., & Bakass, F. (2022). Diffusion test of fertility decline in Arab countries of the Middle East and North Africa (MENA) Region. *Journal of Population and Social Studies [JPSS], 30*, 562–590.
54. Jafari, H., Jaafaripooyan, E., Vedadhir, A. A., Foroushani, A. R., Ahadinejad, B., & Pourreza, A. (2016). Socio-economic factors influencing on total fertility rate in Iran: A panel data analysis for the period of 2002–2012. *Electronic physician, 8*(6), 2551.
55. Götmark, F., & Andersson, M. (2020). Human fertility in relation to education, economy, religion, contraception, and family planning programs. *BMC Public Health, 20*, 1–17.
56. https://blogs.worldbank.org/africacan/7-facts-about-population-in-sub-saharan-africa
57. Veleti, K. (2001). Family structure and its effective influence on fertility. *Journal of Human Ecology, 12*(5), 387–390.
58. Mönkediek, B., & Bras, H. (2018). Family systems and fertility intentions: Exploring the pathways of influence. *European Journal of Population, 34*, 33–57.
59. Chaijaroen, P., & Panda, P. (2023). Women's education, marriage, and fertility outcomes: Evidence from Thailand's compulsory schooling law. *Economics of Education Review, 96*, Article 102440.
60. Nag, A., & Singhal, P. (2013). Impact of education and age at marriage on fertility among Uttar Pradesh migrants of Ludhiana, Punjab, India. *The Anthropologist, 15*(2), 225–230.
61. Khraif, R. M., Salam, A. A., Al-Mutairi, A., Elsegaey, I., & Al Jumaah, A. (2017). Education's impact on fertility: The case of King Saud University women, Riyadh. *Middle East Fertility Society Journal, 22*(2), 125–131.

62. Anita, R., & SDBJG, N. (2010). Prevalence of child marriage and its impact on the fertility and fertility control behaviors of young women in India. *Lancet, 373*(9678), 1883–1889.
63. Tao, P., Coates, R., & Maycock, B. (2012). Investigating marital relationship in infertility: A systematic review of quantitative studies. *Journal of Reproduction & Infertility, 13*(2), 71.
64. Dixit, A., Bhan, N., Benmarhnia, T., Reed, E., Kiene, S. M., Silverman, J., & Raj, A. (2021). The association between early in marriage fertility pressure from in-laws' and family planning behaviors, among married adolescent girls in Bihar and Uttar Pradesh, India. *Reproductive Health, 18*, 1–9.

Chapter 2
Analysis of Human Reproductive Dynamics

2.1 Introduction

The TFR serves as a crucial indicator of human reproductive health, reflecting the average number of children a woman is expected to have during her reproductive years. It offers valuable insights into a population's capacity to achieve desired family sizes while safeguarding overall well-being. Global demographic trends, as indicated by the World Population Prospects, depict a significant decline in TFR, with a projected worldwide fertility rate expected to reach 2.1 births per woman by 2050 [1]. This sharply contrasts with the 1950 average of 5 births per woman, which has steadily declined to 2.3 births per woman in 2021. The magnitude of this shift in birth rates and population dynamics is undeniably noteworthy. Many of the world's most populous countries, such as India, China, and the United States, are notably experiencing a downward trend in fertility rates. Particularly, India has experienced a remarkable 20% decrease in fertility rates per 1000 women over the past decade. The World Bank data presents information on the "crude" birth rate, a demographic indicator that calculates the count of live births in a given population over a particular interval (typically a year) per 1000 people in that population. The term "crude" signifies that this rate is not adjusted for age or other factors, providing a raw count of births relative to the entire population, disregarding age distribution and expressed as "births per 1000 population." The crude birth rate is a valuable metric for gauging the overall fertility level within a population. It offers a broad perspective on birth patterns without considering age-related variations. This metric facilitates comparisons between different regions or periods. Figure 2.1 compares the TFR and CBR among the ten most populous countries worldwide. The findings indicate that seven out of these ten nations have a TFR below the replacement level. This underscores the nuanced interplay between birth rates and TFR, emphasizing their crucial significance in the context of human reproductive health. The TFR emerges as a pivotal factor shaping population dynamics, and a deeper understanding of this correlation contributes to a more comprehensive comprehension of global fertility patterns [2].

KC. Santosh and D. G. Roy, *Artificial Intelligence for Human Fertility: Trends, Insights, and Predictions*, Studies in Computational Intelligence 1230,
https://doi.org/10.1007/978-981-95-1248-5_2

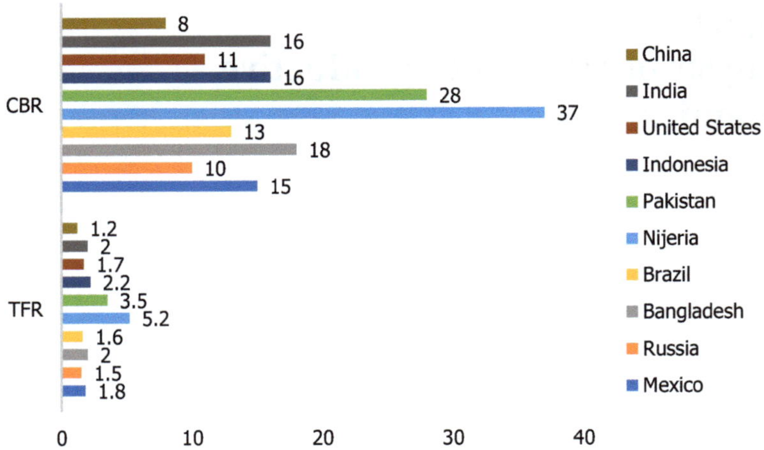

Fig. 2.1 Horizontal bar chart comparing CBR and TFR values across various countries. It includes data for China, India, the United States, Indonesia, Pakistan, Nigeria, Brazil, Bangladesh, Russia, and Mexico [3]. CBR values range from 1 to 37, with Mexico having the highest value. TFR values range from 1.2 to 3.2, with Nigeria having the highest value. A legend on the right associates colours with each country

Reproductive health involves various aspects of physical, mental, and social well-being connected to the human reproductive system and the capacity to have safe and fulfilling sexual experiences. In contrast, fertility refers to an individual's biological capacity to reproduce, with sexual experiences playing a fundamental role in human reproduction. These interconnected factors are pivotal in shaping global population dynamics, birth rates, and TFR [4]. Understanding the techniques employed for assessing human fertility is essential in this context. This assessment involves evaluating an individual or couple's ability to conceive and have children, utilizing various medical and diagnostic tests to identify the underlying causes of fertility issues. The evaluation may encompass factors such as sperm quality, ovulation, fallopian tube health, and uterine condition. Additionally, lifestyle factors, including diet, exercise, and environmental exposures, are also considered as they can significantly impact fertility. These reasons are extended as a cause of impaired fertility [5].

To highlight with greater precision, the ASFR is a critical metric, distinguishing itself from the TFR and CBR. Unlike TFR and BR, ASFR offers a more intricate and nuanced perspective on fertility patterns within a population. Its significance goes beyond the broader insights provided by TFR and BR. ASFR provides additional valuable information on age-related fertility patterns, elucidating how fertility varies among different age groups of women. It also identifies the timing of childbearing, showing whether women tend to have children at an earlier or later age. Furthermore, ASFR plays a pivotal role in identifying fertility trends, reflecting shifts in reproductive behaviour. It is a crucial tool in population projection, contributing to our understanding of future population sizes.

ASFR offers insights into reproductive health by providing a nuanced view of women's reproductive health at various stages of their reproductive years. Integrating ASFR with TFR and crude birth rates allows demographers, policymakers, and researchers to develop a more comprehensive understanding of population growth dynamics [6]. This holistic understanding, in turn, guides targeted interventions and policies aimed at improving reproductive health. Many research articles have been published on this declining rate of ASFR [7]. A study was conducted in Bangladesh to identify the trends of ASFR. They reported decremental ASFR is noticeable in the women's age group [8]. Similarly, a survey was performed to forecast the ASFR of India using different data based on the NHFS rounds. The study outcome replicates a fluctuating ASFR observed in six states of India [9]. Another study was conducted in Uganda to identify the reason for the unchanging fertility rate. They used the data from 2006 to 2016 UDHS and highlighted four factors that affect the ASFR [10]. Finally, the registered data shows the mean childbearing age is related to ASFR. Table 2.1 represents the relationship between TFR, ASFR, and mean childbearing age of 10 populous countries [11]. The data is collected from the United Nations in the World Fertility Data period of 2012.

The data in Table 2.1 indicates that the reference year is within the range of 2007 to 2010. Notably, Fig. 2.1 illustrates a decreasing trend in the TFR in 2021. Specifically, China, which experienced its lowest TFR in 2008, has steadily decreased to a value of 1.2. In contrast, Nigeria, with a TFR of 5.72 in 2007, reported a TFR of 5.2 in 2021. This points to an apparent decline in fertility among the top 10 most populous countries. Given this trend, it becomes crucial to investigate whether this decline is attributable to a preference for lower fertility or if there is a rising prevalence of infertility, thereby uncovering the underlying reasons for this significant shift in fertility rates.

In recent decades, impaired fertility has emerged as a global challenge, characterized by individuals or couples encountering difficulties in achieving pregnancy. This issue constitutes a significant and emotionally challenging barrier within the domain of reproductive health, which is influenced by a range of factors like medical conditions, hormonal imbalances, lifestyle choices, and environmental factors. Impaired fertility often results in extended periods of unsuccessful attempts to conceive, resulting in emotional stress and a far-reaching impact on an individual's overall well-being [12]. Unfortunately, a substantial number of couples worldwide, estimated to be in the range of 60 to 80 million, are confronted with challenges related to impaired fertility or infertility. As per a report by the WHO, one in every four couples in developing countries faces infertility challenges, with a notable concentration of 15 to 20 million affected couples in India alone [13]. In the United States, approximately 6.7 million individuals (about twice the population of Oklahoma) experience difficulties with conception each year, and similar trends of infertility have been reported in other countries over the past decades [14]. Figure 2.2 replicates real-time scenarios depicting infertility cases in the world's most populous countries. Moreover, infertility is common everywhere, and it is rising silently. In addition, these issues are sometimes overlooked or neglected due to a lack of awareness, societal taboos, and sensitivity. However, attention must be paid to identify the

Table 2.1 World's top 10 populous countries ASFR and mean childbearing age

Country	Reference year	TFR	ASFR							Mean age at childbearing*	Source*
			15–19	20–24	25–29	30–34	35–39	40–44	45–49		
Bangladesh	2010	2.32	118	153	107	56	21	6	3	24.7	DHS
Brazil	2008	1.84	71	100	88	64	35	10	1	26.4	NS
China	2008	1.47	5	95	101	54	22	10	7	28.4	NS
India	2010	2.51	37	199	157	66	30	9	4	26.5	NS
Indonesia	2006	2.59	51	135	134	108	65	19	6	28.3	DHS
Pakistan	2007	3.69	16	150	225	173	103	53	18	30.4	NS
Russia	2010	1.57	28	87	95	67	30	6	0	27.5	UNSD
Nigeria	2007	5.72	121	225	265	241	161	87	44	29.8	DHS
Mexico	2008	2.77	87	160	143	99	50	15	2	26.7	UNSD
United States	2008	2.08	41	103	115	99	47	10	1	28.0	UNSD

*Indicates different meanings of each abbreviation
DHS: Signifies that the data are gathered through a Demographic and Health Survey, a program administered by ICF International
NS: Refers to data collected through National Statistics
UNSD: Represents national estimates released by the United Nations Statistics Division
Reference Year: The "Reference year" column represents the middle point of the reference period
Mean Age at Childbearing: The mean age at childbearing represents the average age of mothers at the time of childbirth, if women experience the age-specific fertility rates observed each year throughout their reproductive lives

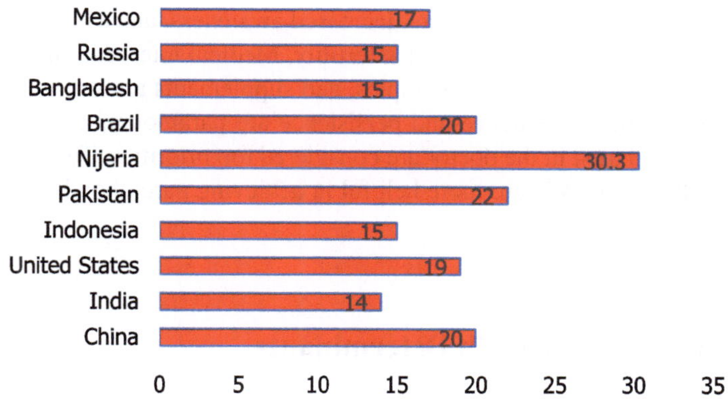

Fig. 2.2 Horizontal bar chart showing the number of people in millions for various countries [16]. China leads with 31 million, followed by India with 21 million, and the United States with 19 million. Other countries include Indonesia, Pakistan, Nigeria, Brazil, Bangladesh, Russia, and Mexico, with values ranging from 1.5 to 30.3 million. Bars are red, and countries are listed on the vertical axis

underlying causes that affect couples, and sometimes an individual's personal life gets hampered. As a result, dissatisfaction occurs, which can lead to isolation, depression, and a sense of hopelessness. Many people may feel embarrassed or hesitant to discuss their struggles openly, and people do not record it as a disease [15].

Breaking the silence on infertility requires normalizing open conversations and creating a more supportive environment. This journey is a rollercoaster of emotions, deeply personal, costly, exhausting, and yet filled with moments of hope. Therefore, raising awareness about infertility is paramount, encompassing its causes, signs, treatments, medications, and more [17]. Once individuals enter this phase, a primary goal is to listen to their partner's perspective, which is essential for inspiring hope. Earlier, infertility was often associated primarily with female factors, leaving male infertility less acknowledged or even neglected [18]. However, in recent decades, male infertility has gained significant attention, with an estimated 30 to 50% of infertility cases being related to male factors. Male infertility can be caused by multiple factors, including testicular dysfunction, hormonal imbalances, lifestyle choices, congenital anatomical abnormalities, exposure to gonadotoxic agents, and aging [19]. Conversely, female factors account for 50% of infertility cases, though the prevalence may vary across different populations. Female infertility has various identified causes [20]. Additionally, other medical conditions can contribute to infertility. It's important to note that infertility is a complex issue rather than a single disease.

Infertility, unlike many diseases, is typically not life-threatening, but it carries a unique and profound emotional impact characterized by complex feelings of grief and loss. This emotional toll can create challenging situations in individuals' lives. Furthermore, infertility is distinct in that its varied causes contribute to its complexity, making it difficult to cure. The prolonged treatment duration often necessitates mental support and psychological counselling for those affected [21]. These differences highlight the need for specialized care, increased awareness, and a holistic approach to tackling the complex challenges of infertility. Medical interventions, changes in life patterns, fertility prevention, therapies, and supplements are ways to overcome infertility. Furthermore, patience and persistence are paramount, and commitment to the process and trust in the doctor are considered top priorities. The most popular procedures, ICSI and IVF, are more helpful in achieving parenthood [22], which is costly and time-consuming.

2.2 Reproductive Health Determinants

In this segment, we are highlighting determinants that impact human reproductive health. According to fertility determinants fall into two categories: background and intermediate or proximate determinants (PD) [23]. The PD of fertility involves a combination of biological and behavioural factors that have a direct impact on fertility. These factors encompass variables such as the age at first marriage, fertility potential, biological factors like *infecundity, contraceptive use, postpartum infertility, abstinence, induced abortion, and sterilization* [24]. The interaction between these biological and behavioural determinants plays a crucial role in shaping and directly affecting fertility levels within populations. Conversely, indirect factors, such as socio-demographic and cultural elements, impact fertility through proximate determinants but in an indirect manner. When an intermediate fertility variable like the *prevalence of contraception shifts*, fertility changes are likely to occur (assuming other intermediate fertility variables remain constant). This contrasts with indirect determinants like *income or education,* where changes may not necessarily lead to immediate fertility alterations [25].

Extensive research has been dedicated to understanding the determinants of reproductive health. A 2011 study, using a descriptive correlational research design conducted between January and April 2006, included 145 randomly selected married women from rural areas in India. The study underscored the significant impact of key determinants on various aspects of women's reproductive health and quality of life, spanning physical, psychological, sexual, family, socio-economic, energy level, and cognitive domains. The assessment of these domains is considered crucial in light of the identified influential determinants [26]. In 2015, a study examined the primary and secondary influences on the reproductive patterns of two distinct groups. The findings suggested that the adoption of contraception, changes in marriage patterns, and induced abortion might contribute to the observed decline in birth rates [27]. In 1978, a study identified a limited set of proximate determinants and developed a straightforward model to quantify their impact on fertility [28]. During the '90s, the relative effects of four proximate determinants were analyzed using data from 12 DHS and WFS of women [25]. Authors in 1984 found that four proximity determinants, including socio-economic, cultural, biological, and environmental factors, play a role in determining fertility [29]. In 2019, a study with a sample size of 16,515 women examined the proximate determinants of fertility, utilizing background variables such as region of residence, educational attainment, wealth index, and place of residence [30]. The impact of proximate determinants on Bangladesh's population has been investigated, with results indicating that contraceptive use and induced abortion play pivotal roles in the country's fertility transition [31]. Among women aged 15 to 49, a study revealed that contraception had the most significant impact on fertility reduction, along with delayed sexual activity/marriage, induced abortion, and childbearing [32]. A demographic survey conducted in 2014 in Bangladesh focused on determinants of fertility, revealing that age at first marriage, spousal age difference, occupation, education, and working status significantly impacted fertility [33]. In 2017, based on survey data (IDHS), determinants of fertility were identified among 1682 women, with results indicating that an increase in education levels contributed to reducing fertility in West Sulawesi [34].

The WHO has highlighted age and lifestyle choices as key contributors to an increased risk of diminished fertility. Numerous research articles have investigated several factors influencing male fertility, encompassing oxidative stress, diet, smoking, metabolic issues, age, occupational exposure, environmental conditions, sperm DNA fragmentation, obesity, and social factors, as well as considering women's sexual satisfaction [35–39]. Similarly, female fertility is influenced by a range of variables, with PCOS recognized as a significant contributor to infertility. Other variables, including tubal abnormalities, polyps, fibroids, ovulatory dysfunction, endometriosis, smoking, psychological distress, lifestyle choices, disrupted sleep patterns, digital inequality, and mobile phone usage, have also been linked to decreased fertility [40–45].

In recent decades, a discernible decline in birth rates has been observed globally, prompting investigations into the impact and extent of the presence of biological factors in this phenomenon. Male factors have emerged as significant contributors, with 40% of male infertility cases categorized as idiopathic, indicating unexplained causes [46]. In this context, environmental and lifestyle factors are observed as crucial conduce to the increasing prevalence of infertility or subfertility in men. A recent study [47] conducted a thorough exploration of the impact of male factors on infertility arising from individual lifestyles. The identified factors include obesity, unhealthy nutrition, physical inactivity, smoking, excessive alcohol intake, psychological stress, exposure to low-level radio-frequency electromagnetic fields (from mobile phones and portable computers), aging, and various other elements. In [48], the researchers investigated the link between dietary patterns and male idiopathic infertility. The findings revealed that environmental factors can indeed influence male fertility. Furthermore, the study concluded that certain nutrients exhibit positive effects, while others can exacerbate fertility issues. In a separate study [49], researchers examined the potential effects of lifestyle factors on male reproductive health. Their findings emphasized that choices such as smoking, alcohol consumption, illicit drug use, obesity, psychological stress, advanced paternal age, dietary habits, and coffee intake can significantly impact male fertility. Furthermore, they identified additional factors, including testicular heat stress, intense cycling training, inadequate sleep, and exposure to electromagnetic radiation from mobile phones, as potential contributors to reproductive health issues. In [50], the authors focused on mitigating male infertility through adjustable lifestyle choices, specifically emphasizing diet, physical activity, and body composition. The findings highlighted that maintaining a balanced dietary fat intake, practicing moderate physical activity, and managing a healthy body composition contribute positively to enhancing semen quality and improving birth outcomes. In [51], the authors acknowledge the importance of environmental and lifestyle factors concerning sperm count and fertility. The study suggests that implementing lifestyle changes, particularly by reducing sedentary time, may negatively impact sperm production. The research outlined in [52] involved the examination of Australian males to elucidate the reasons for unexplained infertility linked to environmental and lifestyle factors. A study involving 1,000 men was conducted to examine the key factors influencing male infertility. The findings suggest that environmental risk factors and lifestyle choices play a substantial role in influencing the likelihood of male infertility. In [53], the researchers carried out a study to investigate sperm DNA fragmentation and its relationship with health, lifestyle, and age-related factors. The results revealed that conditions such as varicocele, impaired glucose tolerance, testicular tumours, smoking, pollution exposure, and paternal age over 50 were associated with the highest levels of sperm DNA fragmentation. In [54], the authors observed a potential impact of both physical activity and sedentary behaviour on the fertility of both women and men. These findings emphasize the necessity for additional investigation in this particular area. In [55], the study explores the potential mechanisms of arsenic toxicity, its adverse effects on male reproductive organs, and its impact on sperm fertility. In [56], a study found that male and female reproductive health is affected due to physiochemical factors. In [57], the authors pointed out that various environmental factors, such as endocrine-disrupting chemicals, heavy metals, air pollution, and electromagnetic fields, can interfere with hormonal regulation through multiple pathways. Therefore, these factors may play a role in male infertility. In [58], the study's authors investigated the influence of the Mediterranean diet on male fertility. The results revealed that embracing a low-carb organic Mediterranean diet was associated with a reduction in sperm DNA fragmentation and an increase in testosterone hormone levels. In [59], a population-based study was carried out to evaluate the effects of cigarette smoking on several factors, such as semen quality, reproductive hormone levels, metabolic profile, and sperm DNA fragmentation.

The referenced studies offer a thorough investigation into the reproductive dynamics of the human body. They underscore specific factors such as *physical inactivity, laptop usage, cigarette smoking, pollution, environmental conditions, tobacco chewing,* and more, emphasizing their pivotal roles in impacting both male and female fertility or reproductive function. Furthermore, engaging in simultaneous exploration will provide valuable insights into gender-specific reproductive metrics.

2.2.1 Proposal 1: Male Measures

A variety of intricate laboratory and radiologic assessments are accessible for the evaluation of male fertility, but these procedures are time-consuming and can impose psychological stress, adding to the global challenge of infertility. The standard approach to male fertility evaluation involves semen analysis, offering essential insights into reproductive health. Criteria such as sperm quality, encompassing motility, morphology, and concentration, play a pivotal role in assessing male fertility [60]. There are several reasons for male infertility, the most important of which are hormonal imbalances, physical issues, sexually transmitted infections, environmental and lifestyle influences, as well as genetic and epigenetic factors. Table 2.2 provides a concise overview of typical male measures associated with human reproduction.

Hormonal defects

The HPG axis plays a crucial role in male reproductive hormone regulation. Comprising the hypothalamus, pituitary gland, and testes, this axis ensures the precise concentration of hormones necessary for male sexual development and function. Any disruptions in this intricate system can lead to infertility [61, 62]. Specifically, the pituitary gland's ability to produce adequate amounts of luteinizing hormone and follicle-stimulating hormone is vital. Insufficient production of these hormones can fail to stimulate the testes, leading to decreased testosterone and sperm production. Conversely, high levels of LH and FSH may be linked to low testosterone levels, which can lead to defects in spermatogenesis. Thus, maintaining the delicate balance within the HPG axis is crucial for proper male reproductive function [63].

Table 2.2 Male measure associated factors

Measures	Key points
Sexual problems	Erectile dysfunction, early ejaculation, and inability to ejaculate
Varicocele	Rising temperature in scrotum, decreased sperm production, and shrinking of testicles
Genetic and epigenetic	Y chromosome and spermatogenesis, genetic disorders, androgen receptor gene mutations, CFTR gene mutations, single nucleotide polymorphisms, hormone receptor gene variations, azoospermia, oligospermia, and abnormalities in seminiferous tubules
Lifestyle habits	Smoking, alcohol consumption, poor diet, overuse of sunbath, prolonged sitting, extremely high temperature, wearing tight clothes, and usage of wi-fi internet
HPG axis (male hormones)	Luteinizing hormone, follicle-stimulating hormone
Physical Infection	Gonorrhea and chlamydia
Environmental toxic	Air pollution, repeated use of drugs such as cocaine and cannabinoids

Physical causes

Various physical issues can disrupt sperm production and hinder the ejaculatory pathway. A common problem is the enlargement of sperm vessels, known as varicocele, affecting around 40% of men [64, 65]. Testicular torsion within the testicular sac can lead to damage due to pressure on sperm vessels and impaired testicular circulation. Chronic and acute genital tract infections are also frequent contributors to male infertility [66]. Mumps viral infection is an additional factor that can lead to testicular atrophy and infertility [67]. Sexually transmitted diseases such as Gonorrhea and Chlamydia can result in male infertility due to epididymal obstruction. In some instances, recurrent ejaculation, where semen is directed into the bladder, constitutes approximately 2% of infertility cases. This condition can stem from anatomical issues with the bladder sphincter [68]. Recognizing and addressing these physical challenges are crucial steps in managing male infertility.

Sexual problems

Numerous sexual issues encompass both physical and psychological aspects. Examples of such problems include erectile dysfunction, also known as impotence, early ejaculation, and the inability to ejaculate [69].

Lifestyle and environmental factors

In general, lifestyle factors affect male reproductive systems in various ways. An unhealthy lifestyle may be one of the greatest reasons, which include smoking, alcohol consumption, and poor diet. Similarly, exposure to hazardous substances in the workplace is common for males. Substances like solvents, insecticides, adhesives, silicones, and radiation can lead to infertility [70–72]. Radiation exposure can result in decreased sperm production, and higher doses of radiation can lead to complete infertility. Overuse of sunbathing, prolonged sitting, extremely high temperatures, wearing tight clothes, and usage of wi-fi internet can harm fertility. Among them, smoking, alcohol consumption, and prolonged sitting are found to be key factors that are associated with progressive degradation in sperm quality [73–75]. Additionally, air pollution and the frequent use of substances like cocaine and cannabinoids are linked to reduced sperm concentration and urinary testosterone levels in men [70]. The influence of lifestyle and environmental factors also alters sperm morphology and negatively impacts sperm motility [76]. Moreover, to identify each factor's relationship, a large number of studies concerned with this aspect are needed.

Genetic and epigenetic factors

Genetic factors contribute to approximately 15% of male infertility and can be categorized into two groups: chromosomal abnormalities and single-gene mutations [77]. Chromosomal abnormalities involve the lack or acquisition of unusual rearrangements in genetic material at the chromosomal level, representing a significant genetic cause of male infertility [78]. These abnormalities can be inherited or acquired. Common genetic causes of male infertility include issues with the Y chromosome and spermatogenesis, genetic disorders, androgen receptor gene mutations, CFTR gene mutations, single-nucleotide polymorphisms, hormone receptor gene variations, azoospermia, oligospermia, and abnormalities in seminiferous tubules. Azoospermia, accounting for about 14% of male infertility cases, is often linked to genetic factors [79, 80]. Additionally, translocations are implicated in 3% of severe oligozoospermia cases [81], and Y chromosome microdeletions are found in 10% of infertile men [82]. Epigenetic factors, such as acetylation and methylation, play a crucial role in modifying gene expression and are implicated in male infertility. Epigenetic dysregulation in sperm from individuals with oligozoospermia and oligoasthenoteratozoospermia has been observed. Furthermore, hypermethylation in several genes is associated with deficiencies in semen parameters and male infertility [83, 84]. Understanding these genetic and epigenetic factors is essential for gaining insight into the complex nature of male infertility and for creating targeted interventions for those affected.

2.2.2 Proposal 2: Female Measures

According to the WHO, several crucial factors contribute to female infertility [85]. The most identified factors include (1) ovulatory disorders, (2) endometriosis, (3) pelvic adhesions, (4) tubal blockage, (5) other tubal/uterine abnormalities, and (6) hyperprolactinemia. Female factors are identified as the cause for approximately 37% of infertile couples. Table 2.3 offers a succinct overview of female measures associated with women's reproductive outcomes.

Table 2.3 Female measure associated factors

Measures	Key points
Anovulation/ovulatory disorder	Hypogonadotropic hypogonadal anovulation, norm gonadotropic norm estrogenic anovulation, hypergonadotropic hypoestrogenic anovulation, hyperprolactinemic anovulation
Pelvic adhesions	Congenital abnormalities, inflammatory diseases, endometriosis, and other pathologies
Hyper-PRL	Both short and long term, encompass menstrual disorders, reduced quality of life, decreased bone mineral density, sexual dysfunction, anovulation, oligomenorrhea, defective ovulation and decreased fertility
Uterine abnormalities	Uterine septum, uterine fibroids, uterine polyps, Asherman's syndrome, and abnormal uterine shape
Endometriosis	Retrograde menstruation, coelomic metaplasia, altered immunity, stem cells, and genetics
Tubal blockage	Congenital abnormalities, inflammatory disease, endometriosis, and other pathologies

(1) Anovulation/ovulatory disorder

Ovulatory disorders account for 25% of the identified causes of female infertility. Ovulation, a key phase of the female menstrual cycle, involves the release of mature eggs (oocytes) from the ovaries. Without the presence of oocytes, fertilization and pregnancy cannot occur. To improve clarity, the WHO has classified ovulatory disorders into four distinct stages:

Hypogonadotropic hypogonadal anovulation

This condition is linked to eating disorders and excessive exercise, which lead to a reduction in hypothalamic GnRH secretion [86]. This, in turn, disrupts the release of key hormones such as FSH and LH. The deficiencies in these hormones result in abnormal follicular development, anovulation, and reduced estrogen levels [87].

Normogonadotropic normoestrogenic anovulation

PCOS is the most prevalent form of normogonadotropic, normoestrogenic anovulation, affecting approximately 80 to 85% of anovulatory patients and 8% of women of reproductive age [88]. Infertility associated with this condition is believed to result from a dysfunction in the development of mature follicles, leading to anovulation. LH levels may be normal or elevated, while FSH and estrogen levels typically remain within normal laboratory ranges [89]. The precise pathophysiology is linked to abnormal pulsatility of GnRH, though the underlying mechanisms of infertility remain poorly understood [90].

Hypergonadotropic hypoestrogenic anovulation

Premature ovarian insufficiency is considered under it, where ovarian resistance is directly related to it. Age is a vital factor that affects women's fertility, and the quality of oocytes declines accordingly. In terms of quantity, a female fetus at 20 weeks' gestation is born with 6 million follicles. It starts decreasing, and at the onset of puberty, the number of follicles is around 3,000,000 [91]. The follicular quantity is affected by smoking, and it is linked to early menopause, particularly in women under the age of 40. Ever-smokers have a more than 30% higher likelihood of experiencing early menopause.

Hyperprolactinemic anovulation

Hyperprolactinemia can result in impaired fertility. Abnormal prolactin secretion is commonly associated with idiopathic hypothalamic dysfunction or the presence of a pituitary adenoma [92]. Furthermore, prolactinoma is recognized as a potential cause of luteal phase defects, which may contribute to infertility [93].

(2) Endometriosis

It is associated with infertility; however, the etiology and pathogenesis remain unclear. Typically, it presents with pain, although 20 to 25% of patients remain asymptomatic. Around 40 to 50% of women experience infertility due to endometriosis [94]. Theories on the etiology of the disease include retrograde menstruation, coelomic metaplasia, altered immunity, stem cells, and genetics [95]. Additionally, it affects gametes and embryos, the fallopian tubes and embryo transport, and the eutopic endometrium; these abnormalities likely all impact fertility [96]. As a result, the lower monthly fecundity rate of approximately 0.02–0.1 is directly associated with a reduced live birth rate [94].

(3) Pelvic adhesions

Approximately 15–20% of cases of female infertility can be attributed to pelvic adhesions [97]. Additionally, 25% of women experience chronic pelvic pain, usually due to adhesions [98]. The common cause of pain is PID, which is caused by sexually transmitted infections (chlamydia and gonorrhea). There are three major causes, such as infection, endometriosis, and pelvic surgery are enumerated. However, all adhesions may not lead to infertility [99]. Conversely, the effect of adhesion is widespread on female reproductive organs like ovaries, fallopian tubes, uterus, and bladder, which often prevent the normal functionality of the reproductive system [100].

(4) Tubal blockage

Obstruction of the fallopian tubes is the most common cause of tubal factor infertility, contributing to 30% to 40% of female fertility issues [85]. Various factors, such as congenital abnormalities, inflammatory diseases, endometriosis, and other pathologies, can lead to partial or complete blockage of the fallopian tubes. Approximately 30% of women facing infertility have issues related to their fallopian tubes, and among them, 10–25% experience proximal fallopian tube obstruction [85]. Managing tubal obstruction involves unblocking the fallopian tubes to restore reproductive function. Detection and diagnostic methods include imaging techniques, hysteroscopy, and laparoscopy [101].

(5) Uterine abnormalities

Most congenital uterine abnormalities are asymptomatic and are often detected incidentally [102]. Conditions such as uterine septum, fibroids, polyps, Asherman's syndrome, and abnormal uterine shapes can have an impact on fertility. In the past, the gold standard for classifying these anomalies involved more invasive procedures. However, imaging modalities including ultrasonography, hysterosalpingography, sonohysterography, and magnetic resonance imaging provide less invasive options for screening [103]. Laparoscopy and hysteroscopy remain reliable methods for accurately classifying uterine anomalies. Additionally, 3D ultrasound has become the preferred diagnostic tool due to its high accuracy, minimally invasive nature, and cost-effectiveness [104].

(6) Hyperprolactinemia (hyper-PRL)

Hyperprolactinemia is a prevalent endocrine disorder affecting both genders across all age groups. The annual incidence is 1.4 per 100,000 persons for men and 8.7 per 100,000 persons for women [105]. While it is a well-established cause of hypothalamic-hypophyseal dysfunction and infertility from a clinical perspective, the underlying mechanisms of these effects remain unclear. The consequences of hyperprolactinemia, both short- and long-term, encompass menstrual disorders, reduced quality of life, decreased bone mineral density, and sexual dysfunction. Common manifestations include anovulation, oligomenorrhea, amenorrhea, and galactorrhea, with defective ovulation and decreased fertility as notable outcomes [106]. In cases of female infertility, PCOS is frequently recognized as a primary contributor to hyperprolactinemia. Numerous studies highlight the significant roles of idiopathic hyperprolactinemia and PCOS in raising prolactin levels, contributing to fertility challenges [107].

2.2.3 Proposal 3: Other Vital Measures

In addition to distinct male and female factors influencing reproductive health, several common factors affect both genders. These are typically regarded as combined factors, contributing directly to reproductive health. These factors encompass age, medications, drug use, obesity, substance use, physical labour, high blood pressure, and physical and psychological stress. Table 2.4 outlines the shared measures that impact the reproductive outcomes of both genders.

Table 2.4 Presentation of common measures for both genders

Measures	Key points
Substance usage	Heavy drinking and consumption of tobacco
Occupational exposure	Women: metals like lead, cadmium, and mercury, pesticides: 1-1-1-trichloroethane, and organic solvents including benzene and toluene, along with ionizing radiation. Men: benzene, whether individually or in combination with toluene and xylene
Physical activity	Swimming, weightlifting, cycling, running
Illicit drugs	Marijuana, cocaine, opioids, methamphetamines, ecstasy, anabolic steroids and lysergic acid diethylamide
Psychological stress	In women, prolonged stress can lead to irregular menstrual cycles or amenorrhea, attributed to stress-induced alterations in the hypothalamus affecting key reproductive hormones
Obesity	Women: affecting ovarian follicular development, the qualitative aspects of oocyte development, fertilization, embryo development, and implantation. Men: sperm concentration, motility, viability, and normal morphology
Age	Females, a natural decline in fecundity typically begins around the age of 32, followed by a substantial decrease, particularly after 37. Advancing male age is associated with prolonged time to conception, reductions in semen quality, and an escalating rate of DNA fragmentation in sperm
Medications	Anti-depressants, calcium channel blockers, alpha-adrenergic blockers, anti-epilepsy drugs and anti-retroviral, are associated with alterations in sperm and pregnancy potential

Age

The relationship between fertility and aging has consistently been intertwined, with the age of the partner remaining the single most crucial factor. In females, a natural decline in fecundity typically begins around the age of 32, followed by a substantial decrease, particularly after the age of 37. This decline is indicative of changes in ovarian reserve, reflecting both the quality and quantity of oocytes affected due to aging [108]. Older women often experience a higher miscarriage rate and an increased incidence of congenital anomalies. Additionally, markers such as serum FSH, basal estradiol levels, antral follicle count, and AMH hormone secretion undergo alterations in this age-related context. In the early 1980s, fertility rates for men in their 30s increased by 21%, and for men aged 40 years and older, the rate surged by nearly 30%. Conversely, the fertility rate for men under 30 years old witnessed a decline of 15% [109]. Advancing male age is associated with prolonged time to conception, reductions in semen quality, and an escalating rate of DNA fragmentation in sperm. Furthermore, there exists a correlation between the age of the male partner and the incidence of birth defects and chromosomal abnormalities [110].

Medications

Pharmaceutical medications can impact both genders, and common medications, including anti-depressants, calcium channel blockers, alpha-adrenergic blockers, anti-epilepsy drugs, and antiretrovirals, are associated with alterations in sperm and pregnancy potential [111]. Anti-depressant medications, frequently used in treating depression, can lead to altered testosterone levels, potentially contributing to male factor infertility. Calcium channel blockers, prescribed for hypertension and heart failure, have been shown to affect sperm motility, contributing to MFI [112]. Alpha-adrenergic blockers, commonly used to treat lower urinary tract symptoms, negatively impact male sperm parameters, including sperm concentration and motility. Additionally, a decrease in ejaculation volume may be observed in 90% of subjects following the use of alpha-adrenergic blockers [113]. Anti-epileptic medications have known side effects on sex hormones, resulting in abnormal sperm morphology, reduced motility, lower sperm count, and decreased testicular volume [114]. High antiretroviral therapy has been associated with serious adverse effects, including reduced sperm motility and abnormal sperm morphology. In women, the widespread use of anti-depressants has been linked to a decrease in natural fertility [115].

Illicit drug usage

The use of illicit drugs, including marijuana, cocaine, opioids, methamphetamines, ecstasy, anabolic steroids, and lysergic acid diethylamide, can have various detrimental effects on human fertility. Marijuana use, for example, has been linked to a decrease in sperm count, motility, and morphology in males, while females may experience disrupted menstrual cycles and ovulation, impacting fertility for both genders [116]. Cocaine use is associated with alterations in sperm, and women who use cocaine commonly experience ovulatory dysfunction, further affecting fertility [117]. Opioid use can lead to hormonal imbalances, negatively impacting sperm production and quality [118]. Numerous studies have suggested that the use of illicit drugs has overall effects on male seminal parameters, while women may commonly experience menstrual complexities. Both factors are crucial considerations for individuals seeking to achieve pregnancy [119].

Obesity

It can contribute to infertility through various pathways, affecting ovarian follicular development, the qualitative and quantitative aspects of oocyte development, fertilization, embryo development, and implantation. Numerous studies have demonstrated a higher prevalence of anovulatory infertility in overweight and obese individuals [120]. In overweight and obese women, menstrual disturbances are four times more common, and these disturbances are associated with infertility. Additionally, obesity and its underlying mechanisms have a detrimental impact on semen parameters in men, including sperm concentration, motility, viability, and normal morphology. Furthermore, obesity inhibits chromatin condensation and contributes to DNA fragmentation, increased apoptosis, and epigenetic changes, which can be passed on to the offspring [121].

Substance usage

This encompasses smoking tobacco, using other tobacco products, and engaging in heavy drinking. Smoking is listed among the risk factors for over 60% of noncommunicable diseases, and each year, more than six million deaths are attributed to substance consumption (tobacco) and second-hand smoke [122]. Recent reports from the WHO confirm that smoking has a detrimental impact on human fertility. Approximately 30% of women of reproductive age who smoke cigarettes experience impaired fertility, with nicotine, cotinine, and cadmium identified as potential culprits that reduce creatine kinase activity in sperm [123].

Occupational exposure

Occupational exposure presents a spectrum of risks to human fertility, arising from exposure to a variety of chemical, physical, biological, and occupational factors. Current data indicate that the impact of these factors on female fertility is limited compared to their effects on males. Specific toxicants, such as metals like lead, cadmium, and mercury, pesticides like (4-chlorophenyl)-1,1,1-trichloroethane, and organic solvents including benzene and toluene, along with ionizing radiation, have been linked to adverse effects on the female reproductive system. These effects can manifest either directly or indirectly through hormonal disruptions, molecular changes, oxidative stress, and DNA methylation, influencing fertility, pregnancy, and their outcomes [124]. Concerning male fertility, a noteworthy decline in semen quality has been observed. Studies indicate that exposure to benzene, whether individually or in combination with toluene and xylene, is associated with elevated benzene levels in both blood and seminal plasma. Such exposure has been correlated with significant genome damage, abnormal sperm count, motility issues, morphological abnormalities, as well as disomy X, Y, and hyperhaploidy, even at low levels [125, 126].

Psychological stress

Recent research, highlighted in a comprehensive review, emphasizes the intricate connection between emotional stress and fertility, particularly in women [127]. Chronic stress significantly disrupts the delicate hormonal balance crucial for fertility in both women and men. In women, prolonged stress can lead to irregular menstrual cycles or amenorrhea, attributed to stress-induced alterations in the hypothalamus affecting key reproductive hormones. The intricate interplay between stress hormones like cortisol and sex hormones such as estrogen and progesterone can modify ovulation patterns, diminishing the likelihood of successful conception. Additionally, stress-related psychological factors may contribute to a decline in sexual desire and intimacy, introducing further complexity. Persistent stress in women navigating pregnancy heightens the risk of complications, including preterm birth and low birth weight [128]. Similarly, in men, stress-induced elevation of cortisol levels disrupts the delicate hormonal balance, negatively impacting testosterone production and influencing various aspects of sperm quality, including count, motility, and morphology. Chronic stress in men may also contribute to sexual difficulties such as erectile dysfunction and diminished libido [129].

Physical activity

The American Society for Reproductive Medicine offers clear guidance on the effects of smoking, alcohol consumption, and diet on conception. However, there is a noticeable absence of specific recommendations regarding patient involvement in physical activity and exercise. A recent study suggests that in women with low energy status due to a high physical activity workload, reproduction is often delayed, slowed, or temporarily compromised [130]. Conversely, enhancing women's energy status through the introduction of work-saving technologies has been demonstrated to frequently increase fertility [131]. Concerning men, the literature provides diverse findings regarding the impact of physical activity on semen quality. Common activities among men, such as swimming, racquet sports, running, cycling, and weightlifting, show varied effects. A study indicates that moderate-intensity swimming effectively mitigated the deleterious effects of elevated oxidative stress [132]. However, it is essential to note that testicular spermatogenic cells exhibited increased DNA damage induced by swimming, and weightlifters displayed lower sperm concentration and total sperm counts compared to men who did not engage in regular exercise [133]. Conversely, when examining specific types of PA like biking, an association was identified, suggesting that biking for more than 5 h per week was linked to lower sperm concentration and low total motile sperm compared to those with no regular activity.

2.3 Prevention and Diagnosis

Reproductive health encompasses the prevention and management of various issues, including infertility, conception, and pregnancy. Individuals can promote their reproductive health by increasing social awareness, acquiring comprehensive knowledge, practicing family planning, and seeking guidance from physicians. While natural conception is a straightforward process, artificial conception can be time-consuming, expensive, and may impose psychological burdens. Infertility, affecting 60 to 80 million couples and 186 million individuals, presents a significant challenge. Despite its widespread impact, infertility is often not officially classified as a disease due to its less symptomatic nature. This characteristic often leads individuals to seek medical assistance only at advanced stages, contributing to heightened levels of depression and anxiety.

Hence, to mitigate these effects, preventive measures include the use of appropriate medications, adopting a healthy diet, engaging in regular physical activity, maintaining a suitable body weight, addressing trends in delayed marriage, ensuring regular menstrual cycles, and discouraging late marriage. On the other hand, the diagnostic process involves clinical examinations, blood tests, ultrasound scans, ovulation testing, and more. Following a diagnosis, healthcare professionals establish a treatment protocol based on the nature and severity of the condition. The decision between invasive and non-invasive treatments is contingent on factors such as the specific diagnosis, overall health, and treatment objectives.

Non-invasive fertility treatments focus on improving fertility without the use of tools, incorporating lifestyle modifications, ovulation tracking, supplements, stress reduction, dietary changes, and timed intercourse. On the other hand, invasive treatments encompass Assisted Reproductive Technologies like Intrauterine Insemination, Intracytoplasmic Sperm Injection, In Vitro Fertilization, as well as procedures such as laparoscopy, assisted hatching, embryo cryopreservation, freezing, egg freezing, and tubal ligation reversal. These invasive treatments are associated with significant costs, and their success rates depend on several factors, necessitating careful consideration. Ultimately, physicians play a pivotal role not just in diagnosing and treating conditions but also in providing guidance on disease prevention. The emphasis on prevention underscores its greater benefits compared to cure, underscoring its significant impact on overall patient health in contemporary society.

2.4 Conclusion

Reproductive measures provide reliable benchmarks for evaluating factors that influence human fertility, addressing aspects related to females, males, and other contributing elements. A closer examination reveals that while some measures strongly correlate with clinician-related factors, others are modifiable and can indirectly affect fertility or the reproductive system. Over the past two decades, infertility rates have risen noticeably, often without clear clinical explanations, posing a significant challenge. However, establishing a definitive cause-and-effect relationship remains difficult, primarily due to the lack of objective assessment tools or standardized measures.

References

1. https://desapublications.un.org/file/989/download. Last accessed: 4.10.23.
2. https://www.who.int/data/gho/indicator-metadata-registry/imr-details/3344. Last accessed: 5/10/23.
3. https://data.worldbank.org/. Last accessed: 10/12/23.
4. https://www.who.int/southeastasia/health-topics/reproductive-health. Last accessed: 6/12/23.
5. Crawford, S., Smith, R. A., Kuwabara, S. A., & Grigorescu, V. (2017). Risks factors and treatment use related to infertility and impaired fecundity among reproductive-aged women. *Journal of Women's Health, 26*(5), 500–510.
6. Ghaem, H., Zare, M., Hemmati, A., Moghadami, M., Moradi, F., & Semati, A. (2019). Pattern of changes in age-specific fertility rates, total fertility rate, and cohort fertility rate in rural areas of Fars Province, Southern Iran (1988–2012). *Journal of Family & Reproductive Health, 13*(1), 1.
7. Pittenger, D. B. (1980). Some models of age-specific fertility rates. *Environment and Planning A, 12*(10), 1145–1164.
8. Fazle Rabbi, A. M., & Kabir, M. (2015). Explaining fertility transition of a developing country: An analysis of quantum and tempo effect. *Fertility Research and Practice, 1*, 1–6.
9. Srivastava, U., Singh, K. K., Pandey, A., & Narayan, N. (2021). Experiments in modeling recent Indian fertility pattern. *Scientific Reports, 11*(1), 6592.
10. Ariho, P., & Kabagenyi, A. (2020). Age at first marriage, age at first sex, family size preferences, contraception and change in fertility among women in Uganda: Analysis of the 2006–2016 period. *BMC Women's Health, 20*, 1–13.
11. https://data.un.org/documentdata.aspx?id=319. Last accessed: 6/12/23.
12. Simionescu, G., Doroftei, B., Maftei, R., Obreja, B. E., Anton, E., Grab, D., Ilea, C., & Anton, C. (2021). The complex relationship between infertility and psychological distress (review). *Experimental and Therapeutic Medicine, 21*(4), 306. https://doi.org/10.3892/etm.2021.9737
13. Katole, A., & Saoji, A. V. (2019). Prevalence of primary infertility and its associated risk factors in urban population of Central India: A community-based cross-sectional study. *Indian Journal of community medicine: Official Publication of Indian Association of Preventive & Social Medicine, 44*(4), 337–341. https://doi.org/10.4103/ijcm.IJCM_7_19
14. Stephen, E. H., & Chandra, A. (2006). Declining estimates of infertility in the United States: 1982–2002. *Fertility and Sterility, 86*(3), 516–523.
15. Xie, Y., Ren, Y., Niu, C., Zheng, Y., Yu, P., & Li, L. (2023). The impact of stigma on mental health and quality of life of infertile women: A systematic review. *Frontiers in Psychology, 13*, 1093459. https://doi.org/10.3389/fpsyg.2022.1093459
16. https://worldpopulationreview.com/country-rankings/total-fertility-rate. Last accessed: 14/12/23.
17. Singh, V., Rajpal, G., Majumdar, S., Mandal, S., & Sahu, R. (2023). Awareness, knowledge, and psycho-emotional aspect of infertility among women seeking fertility assistance at a tertiary care hospital in Chhattisgarh, a cross-sectional study. *Journal of Education and Health Promotion, 12*, 3. https://doi.org/10.4103/jehp.jehp_581_22

18. Kim, M., Yi, S. J., & Hong, J. E. (2020). Experiences of women with male factor infertility under in vitro fertilization. *International Journal of Environmental Research and Public Health, 17*(21), 7809. https://doi.org/10.3390/ijerph17217809
19. Eisenberg, M. L., Esteves, S. C., Lamb, D. J., Hotaling, J. M., Giwercman, A., Hwang, K., & Cheng, Y. S. (2023). Male infertility. *Nature Reviews. Disease Primers, 9*(1), 49. https://doi.org/10.1038/s41572-023-00459-w
20. Agarwal, A., Mulgund, A., Hamada, A., & Chyatte, M. R. (2015). A unique view on male infertility around the globe. *Reproductive Biology and Endocrinology: RB&E, 13*, 37. https://doi.org/10.1186/s12958-015-0032-1
21. Jain, M., & Singh, M. (2022). Assisted reproductive technology (ART) techniques. In *StatPearls [Internet]*. StatPearls Publishing.
22. Boulet, S. L., Chandra, A., Rosen, A., & De Cherney, A. (2019). Infertility and ART. *Assisted Reproductive Technology Surveillance*, 1–11.
23. Ahmed, S. S. (2020). Roles of proximate determinants of fertility in recent fertility decline in Ethiopia: Application of the revised Bongaarts model. *Open Access Journal of Contraception, 11*, 33–41. https://doi.org/10.2147/OAJC.S251693
24. Ahmed, K. J., Tan, Y., & Rudd, D. (2024). Exploring the relationship between changes in fertility and disasters: A review of the literature. *Journal of Population Research, 41*(1), 1–29.
25. Jolly, C. L., & Gribble, J. N. (1993). The proximate determinants of fertility. In *Demographic change in sub-Saharan Africa* (pp. 68–116).
26. Stumbar, S. E., Garba, N. A., & Holder, C. (2018). Let's talk about sex: The social determinants of sexual and reproductive health for second-year medical students. *MedEdPORTAL: The Journal of Teaching and Learning Resources, 14*, 10772. https://doi.org/10.15766/mep_2374-8265.10772
27. D'souza, M. S., Somayaji, G., & Subrahmanya Nairy, K. (2011). Determinants of reproductive health and related quality of life among Indian women in mining communities. *Journal of Advanced Nursing, 67*(9), 1963–1975.
28. Bongaarts, J. (2015). Modeling the fertility impact of the proximate determinants: Time for a tune-up. *Demographic Research, 33*, 535–560.
29. Bongaarts, J., Frank, O., & Lesthaeghe, R. (1984). The proximate determinants of fertility in sub-Saharan Africa. *Population and Development Review*, 511–537.
30. Laelago, T., Habtu, Y., & Yohannes, S. (2019). Proximate determinants of fertility in Ethiopia; an application of revised Bongaarts model. *Reproductive Health, 16*, 1–9.
31. Rahman, M. M. (2020). Role of proximate determinants in recent and past fertility stalls in Bangladesh. *Biodemography and Social Biology, 65*(2), 119–136.
32. Chemhaka, G. B., & Odimegwu, C. O. (2019). The proximate determinants of fertility in Eswatini. *African Journal of Reproductive Health, 23*(2), 65–75.
33. Nahar, M. Z., & Zahangir, M. S. (2019). Determinants of fertility in Bangladesh: Evidence from the 2014 demographic and health survey. *International Quarterly of Community Health Education, 40*(1), 29–35.
34. Muslimin, I., Hamzah, H., Rahman, K., Sukardi, S., & Akbar, F. (2022). Determinants of fertility in West Sulawesi Province further analysis of Indonesia health demography survey data (IDHS) 2017. *Indonesian Journal of Global Health Research, 4*(4), 969–974.
35. Bala, R., Singh, V., Rajender, S., & Singh, K. (2021). Environment, lifestyle, and female infertility. *Reproductive Sciences, 28*, 617–638.
36. Sharpe, R. M., & Franks, S. (2002). Environment, lifestyle and infertility—An inter-generational issue. *Nature Medicine, 8*(Suppl 10), S33–S40.
37. Sudhakaran, G., Kesavan, D., Kandaswamy, K., Guru, A., & Arockiaraj, J. (2024). Unravelling the epigenetic impact: oxidative stress and its role in male infertility-associated sperm dysfunction. *Reproductive Toxicology*, 108531.
38. Stoop, D., Cobo, A., & Silber, S. (2014). Fertility preservation for age-related fertility decline. *The Lancet, 384*(9950), 1311–1319.
39. Best, D., & Bhattacharya, S. (2015). Obesity and fertility. *Hormone Molecular Biology and Clinical Investigation, 24*(1), 5–10.

40. Billari, F. C., Rotondi, V., & Trinitapoli, J. (2020). Mobile phones, digital inequality, and fertility. *Demographic Research, 42*, 1057–1096.
41. Maggiore, U. L. R., Chiappa, V., Ceccaroni, M., Roviglione, G., Savelli, L., Ferrero, S., Raspagliesi, F., & Bascio, L. S. (2024). Epidemiology of infertility in women with endometriosis. *Best Practice & Research Clinical Obstetrics & Gynaecology*, 102454.
42. Tao, L., Wang, Q., Zeng, X., Fu, L., Li, J., & Chen, H. (2024). Psychological distress in adult women of reproductive age at different stages after breast cancer diagnosis: A qualitative study. *Journal of Clinical Nursing*.
43. Zuberi, N. F., & Batool, S. (2024). Polycystic ovary syndrome and subfertility: Ovulation dysregulation and fertility problems (clinical features and pathophysiology). In *Polycystic ovary syndrome* (pp. 51–55). Elsevier.
44. Carranza-Mamane, B., Havelock, J., Hemmings, R., Cheung, A., Sierra, S., Case, A., Dwyer, C., Graham, J., Liu, K., Murdock, W., Vause, T., Wong, B., & Burnett, M. (2015). The management of uterine fibroids in women with otherwise unexplained infertility. *Journal of Obstetrics and Gynaecology Canada, 37*(3), 277–285.
45. Al Chami, A., & Saridogan, E. (2017). Endometrial polyps and subfertility. *The Journal of Obstetrics and Gynecology of India, 67*, 9–14.
46. Ortac, M. S., Hacioglu, A., Uludag, S. Z., Karaca, Z., Unluhizarci, K., Kelestimur, F., & Tanriverdi, F. (2024). Evaluation of growth hormone deficiency in women with unexplained infertility. *Growth Hormone & IGF Research*, 101571.
47. Corsini, C., Boeri, L., Candela, L., Pozzi, E., Belladelli, F., Capogrosso, P., Fallara, G., Schifano, N., Cignoli, D., Ventimiglia, E., D'Arma, A., Alfano, M., Montorsi, F., & Salonia, A. (2023). Is there a relevant clinical impact in differentiating idiopathic versus unexplained male infertility? *The World Journal of Men's Health, 41*(2), 354.
48. Cargnelutti, F., Pallotti, F., Carlini, T., Faja, F., Vestri, A.R., Fegatelli, D.A., Lenzi, A., Lombardo, F., & Paoli, D. (2023). A decade of WHO 2010: Total sperm number temporal trend and role of lifestyle factors. *Asian Journal of Andrology*, 10–4103.
49. Durairajanayagam, D. (2018). Lifestyle causes of male infertility. *Arab Journal of Urology, 16*(1), 10–20.
50. Hayden, R. P., Flannigan, R., & Schlegel, P. N. (2018). The role of lifestyle in male infertility: Diet, physical activity, and body habitus. *Current Urology Reports, 19*, 1–10.
51. Sharpe, R. M. (2000). Environment, lifestyle and male infertility. *Best Practice & Research Clinical Endocrinology & Metabolism, 14*(3), 489–503.
52. Biggs, S. N., Kennedy, J., Lewis, S. L., Hearps, S., O'Bryan, M. K., McLachlan, R., von Saldern, S., Chambers, G., & Halliday, J. (2023). Lifestyle and environmental risk factors for unexplained male infertility: study protocol for Australian Male Infertility Exposure (AMIE), a case–control study. *Reproductive Health, 20*(1), 1–9.
53. Szabó, A., Váncsa, S., Hegyi, P., Váradi, A., Forintos, A., Filipov, T., Acs, J., Acs, N., Szarvas, T., Nyirady, P., & Kopa, Z. (2023). Lifestyle-, environmental-, and additional health factors associated with an increased sperm DNA fragmentation: a systematic review and meta-analysis. *Reproductive Biology and Endocrinology, 21*(1), 5.
54. Du, C., & Tuo, Y. (2023). Correlation of DNA fragments with routine semen parameters and lifestyle and their impact on assisted reproductive outcomes. *Revista Internacional de Andrología, 21*(2), Article 100337.
55. Brinson, A. K., da Silva, S. G., Hesketh, K. R., & Evenson, K. R. (2023). Impact of physical activity and sedentary behavior on spontaneous female and male fertility: A systematic review. *Journal of Physical Activity and Health, 20*(7), 600–615.
56. Ramezanifar, S., Beyrami, S., Mehrifar, Y., Ramezanifar, E., Soltanpour, Z., Namdari, M., & Gharari, N. (2023). Occupational exposure to physical and chemical risk factors: A systematic review of reproductive pathophysiological effects in women and men. *Safety and Health at Work, 14*(1), 17–30.
57. Pallotti, F., Pelloni, M., Colangelo, S., Gianfrilli, D., Lenzi, A., Lombardo, F., & Paoli, D. (2023). Environmental impact on semen quality and male fertility. In *Environmental endocrinology and endocrine disruptors: Endocrine and endocrine-targeted actions and related human diseases* (pp. 239–269).

58. Corsetti, V., Notari, T., & Montano, L. (2023). Effects of the low-carb organic Mediterranean diet on testosterone levels and sperm DNA fragmentation. *Current Research in Food Science*, 100636.
59. Osadchuk, L., Kleshchev, M., & Osadchuk, A. (2023). Effects of cigarette smoking on semen quality, reproductive hormone levels, metabolic profile, zinc and sperm DNA fragmentation in men: Results from a population-based study. *Frontiers in Endocrinology, 14.*
60. Vasan, S. S. (2011). Semen analysis and sperm function tests: How much to test? *Indian Journal of Urology: IJU : Journal of the Urological Society of India, 27*(1), 41–48. https://doi.org/10.4103/0970-1591.78424
61. Achermann, J. C., & Jameson, J. L. (1999). Fertility and infertility: Genetic contributions from the hypothalamic-pituitary-gonadal axis. *Molecular Endocrinology, 13*(6), 812–818.
62. Caroppo, E. (2009). Male hypothalamic-pituitary-gonadal axis. In *Infertility in the male* (pp. 14–28). Cambridge University.
63. Oduwole, O. O., Huhtaniemi, I. T., & Misrahi, M. (2021). The roles of luteinizing hormone, follicle-stimulating hormone and testosterone in spermatogenesis and folliculogenesis revisited. *International Journal of Molecular Sciences, 22*(23), 12735. https://doi.org/10.3390/ijms222312735
64. Kantartzi, P. D., Goulis, C.hD., Goulis, G. D., & Papadimas, I. (2007). Male infertility and varicocele: myths and reality. *Hippokratia, 11*(3), 99–104.
65. Maheshwari, A., Muneer, A., Lucky, M., Mathur, R., McEleny, K., & British Association of Urological Surgeons and the British Fertility Society. (2022). A review of varicocele treatment and fertility outcomes. *Human Fertility, 25*(2), 209–216.
66. Schuppe, H. C., Pilatz, A., Hossain, H., Diemer, T., Wagenlehner, F., & Weidner, W. (2017). Urogenital infection as a risk factor for male infertility. *Deutsches Arzteblatt International, 114*(19), 339–346. https://doi.org/10.3238/arztebl.2017.0339
67. Wu, H., Wang, F., Tang, D., & Han, D. (2021). Mumps Orchitis: Clinical aspects and mechanisms. *Frontiers in Immunology, 12,* Article 582946. https://doi.org/10.3389/fimmu.2021.582946
68. Fode, M., Krogh-Jespersen, S., Brackett, N. L., Ohl, D. A., Lynne, C. M., & Sønksen, J. (2012). Male sexual dysfunction and infertility associated with neurological disorders. *Asian Journal of Andrology, 14*(1), 61–68. https://doi.org/10.1038/aja.2011.70
69. Corona, G. (2022). Erectile dysfunction and premature ejaculation: A continuum movens supporting couple sexual dysfunction. *Journal of Endocrinological Investigation, 45*(11), 2029–2041. https://doi.org/10.1007/s40618-022-01793-8
70. Babakhanzadeh, E., Nazari, M., Ghasemifar, S., & Khodadadian, A. (2020). Some of the factors involved in male infertility: A prospective review. *International Journal of General Medicine, 13,* 29–41. https://doi.org/10.2147/IJGM.S241099
71. Padrão, P., Lunet, N., Santos, A. C., & Barros, H. (2007). Smoking, alcohol, and dietary choices: Evidence from the Portuguese National Health Survey. *BMC Public Health, 7,* 138. https://doi.org/10.1186/1471-2458-7-138
72. Kesari, K. K., Agarwal, A., & Henkel, R. (2018). Radiations and male fertility. *Reproductive Biology and Endocrinology: RB&E, 16*(1), 118. https://doi.org/10.1186/s12958-018-0431-1
73. Yildirim, M. E., Kaynar, M., Badem, H., Cavis, M., Karatas, O. F., & Cimentepe, E. (2015). What is harmful for male fertility: Cell phone or the wireless Internet? *The Kaohsiung Journal of Medical Sciences, 31*(9), 480–484.
74. Mínguez-Alarcón, L., Gaskins, A. J., Chiu, Y. H., Messerlian, C., Williams, P. L., Ford, J. B., Souter, I., Hauser, R., & Chavarro, J. E. (2018). Type of underwear worn and markers of testicular function among men attending a fertility center. *Human Reproduction (Oxford, England), 33*(9), 1749–1756. https://doi.org/10.1093/humrep/dey259
75. Takahashi, M. (2011). Heat stress on reproductive function and fertility in mammals. *Reproductive Medicine and Biology, 11*(1), 37–47. https://doi.org/10.1007/s12522-011-0105-6
76. Durairajanayagam, D. (2018). Lifestyle causes of male infertility. *Arab Journal of Urology, 16*(1), 10–20. https://doi.org/10.1016/j.aju.2017.12.004

77. Alshaya, D. S. (2022). Genetic and epigenetic factors associated with depression: An updated overview. *Saudi Journal of Biological Sciences, 29*(8), Article 103311. https://doi.org/10.1016/j.sjbs.2022.103311
78. Harton, G. L., & Tempest, H. G. (2012). Chromosomal disorders and male infertility. *Asian Journal of Andrology, 14*(1), 32–39. https://doi.org/10.1038/aja.2011.66
79. Dohle, G. R., Halley, D. J. J., Van Hemel, J. O., Van Den Ouwel, A. M. W., Pieters, M. H. E. C., Weber, R. F. A., & Govaerts, L. C. P. (2002). Genetic risk factors in infertile men with severe oligozoospermia and azoospermia. *Human Reproduction, 17*(1), 13–16.
80. Colaco, S., & Modi, D. (2018). Genetics of the human Y chromosome and its association with male infertility. *Reproductive Biology and Endocrinology, 16*, 1–24.
81. Kim, S. Y., Kim, H. J., Lee, B. Y., Park, S. Y., Lee, H. S., & Seo, J. T. (2017). Y chromosome microdeletions in infertile men with non-obstructive azoospermia and severe Oligozoospermia. *Journal of Reproduction & Infertility, 18*(3), 307–315.
82. Denomme, M. M., McCallie, B. R., Parks, J. C., Booher, K., Schoolcraft, W. B., & Katz-Jaffe, M. G. (2018). Inheritance of epigenetic dysregulation from male factor infertility has a direct impact on reproductive potential. *Fertility and Sterility, 110*(3), 419–428.
83. Mahmmod, H. G., & Ali, A. M. (2023). Effect of sperm global methylation level on sperm parameter. *History of Medicine, 9*(1), 2472–2477.
84. Shamsi, M. B., Kumar, K., & Dada, R. (2011). Genetic and epigenetic factors: Role in male infertility. *Indian Journal of Urology: IJU: Journal of the Urological Society of India, 27*(1), 110.
85. Ambildhuke, K., Pajai, S., Chimegave, A., Mundhada, R., & Kabra, P. (2022). A review of tubal factors affecting fertility and its management. *Cureus, 14*(11), Article e30990. https://doi.org/10.7759/cureus.30990
86. Santoro, N., Filicori, M., & Crowley, W. F., Jr. (1986). Hypogonadotropic disorders in men and women: Diagnosis and therapy with pulsatile gonadotropin-releasing hormone. *Endocrine Reviews, 7*(1), 11–23. https://doi.org/10.1210/edrv-7-1-11
87. Perkins, R. B., Hall, J. E., & Martin, K. A. (1999). Neuroendocrine abnormalities in hypothalamic amenorrhea: Spectrum, stability, and response to neurotransmitter modulation. *The Journal of Clinical Endocrinology and Metabolism, 84*(6), 1905–1911. https://doi.org/10.1210/jcem.84.6.5823
88. Hull, M. G. (1987). Epidemiology of infertility and polycystic ovarian disease: Endocrinological and demographic studies. *Gynecological Endocrinology: The Official Journal of the International Society of Gynecological Endocrinology, 1*(3), 235–245. https://doi.org/10.3109/09513598709023610
89. Rotterdam ESHRE/ASRM-Sponsored PCOS consensus workshop group. (2004). Revised 2003 consensus on diagnostic criteria and long-term health risks related to polycystic ovary syndrome (PCOS). *Human Reproduction (Oxford, England), 19*(1), 41–47. https://doi.org/10.1093/humrep/deh098
90. Fauser, B. C., & Van Heusden, A. M. (1997). Manipulation of human ovarian function: Physiological concepts and clinical consequences. *Endocrine Reviews, 18*(1), 71–106. https://doi.org/10.1210/edrv.18.1.0290
91. Baker, T. G. (1971). Radiosensitivity of mammalian oocytes with particular reference to the human female. *American Journal of Obstetrics and Gynecology, 110*(5), 746–761. https://doi.org/10.1016/0002-9378(71)90271-7
92. Infertility Workup for the Women's Health Specialist. (2019). ACOG committee opinion, number 781. *Obstetrics and Gynecology, 133*(6), e377–e384. https://doi.org/10.1097/AOG.0000000000003271
93. Seppälä, M., Ranta, T., & Hirvonen, E. (1976). Hyperprolactinaemia and luteal insufficiency. *Lancet (London, England), 1*(7953), 229–230. https://doi.org/10.1016/s0140-6736(76)91343-x
94. Bulletti, C., Coccia, M. E., Battistoni, S., & Borini, A. (2010). Endometriosis and infertility. *Journal of Assisted Reproduction and Genetics, 27*(8), 441–447. https://doi.org/10.1007/s10815-010-9436-1

95. Prescott, J., Farland, L. V., Tobias, D. K., Gaskins, A. J., Spiegelman, D., Chavarro, J. E., Rich-Edwards, J. W., Barbieri, R. L., & Missmer, S. A. (2016). A prospective cohort study of endometriosis and subsequent risk of infertility. *Human Reproduction (Oxford, England), 31*(7), 1475–1482. https://doi.org/10.1093/humrep/dew085
96. Macer, M. L., & Taylor, H. S. (2012). Endometriosis and infertility: A review of the pathogenesis and treatment of endometriosis-associated infertility. *Obstetrics and Gynecology Clinics of North America, 39*(4), 535–549. https://doi.org/10.1016/j.ogc.2012.10.002
97. Ghobrial, S., Ott, J., & Parry, J. P. (2023). An overview of postoperative intraabdominal adhesions and their role on female infertility: A narrative review. *Journal of Clinical Medicine, 12*(6), 2263. https://doi.org/10.3390/jcm12062263
98. Fehring, R. J., Bouchard, T., & Meyers, M. (2018). Influence of contraception use on the reproductive health of adolescents and young adults. *The Linacre Quarterly, 85*(2), 167–177.
99. Diamond, E. (1979). Lysis of postoperative pelvic adhesions in infertility. *Obstetrical & Gynecological Survey, 34*(8), 621–622.
100. Schlafer, D. H., & Foster, R. A. (2016). Female genital system. *Jubb, Kennedy & Palmer's Pathology of Domestic Animals, 3*, 358.
101. Varlas, V., Rhazi, Y., Cloțea, E., Borș, R. G., Mirică, R. M., & Bacalbașa, N. (2021). Hysterolaparoscopy: A gold standard for diagnosing and treating infertility and benign uterine pathology. *Journal of Clinical Medicine, 10*(16), 3749. https://doi.org/10.3390/jcm10163749
102. Jayaprakasan, K., & Ojha, K. (2022). Diagnosis of congenital uterine abnormalities: Practical considerations. *Journal of Clinical Medicine, 11*(5), 1251. https://doi.org/10.3390/jcm11051251
103. Alcázar, J. L., Carriles, I., Cajas, M. B., Costa, S., Fabra, S., Cabrero, M., Castro, E., Tomaizeh, A., Laza, M. V., Monroy, A., Martinez, I., Aguilar, M. I., Hernani, E., Castellet, C., Oliva, A., Pascual, M. Á., & Guerriero, S. (2023). Diagnostic performance of two-dimensional ultrasound, two-dimensional sonohysterography and three-dimensional ultrasound in the diagnosis of septate uterus-A systematic review and meta-analysis. *Diagnostics (Basel, Switzerland), 13*(4), 807. https://doi.org/10.3390/diagnostics13040807
104. Kupesic, S. (2001). Clinical implications of sonographic detection of uterine anomalies for reproductive outcome. *Ultrasound in Obstetrics and Gynecology: The Official Journal of the International Society of Ultrasound in Obstetrics and Gynecology, 18*(4), 387–400.
105. Dehghan, E., Namiranian, N., Ghadiri-Anari, A., Kazem Razavi Ratki, S., & Azizi, R. (2022). Evaluation of hyperprolactinemia risk factors in infertile women referred to Yazd Infertility Center: A cross-sectional study. *International Journal of Reproductive Biomedicine, 19*(12), 1085–1090. https://doi.org/10.18502/ijrm.v19i12.10059
106. Kostrzak, A., & Męczekalski, B. (2015). Wpływ hiperprolaktynemii na gęstość mineralną kości [Hyperprolactinaemia and bone mineral density]. *Polski merkuriusz lekarski: Organ Polskiego Towarzystwa Lekarskiego, 39*(230), 122–125.
107. Davoudi, Z., Araghi, F., Vahedi, M., Mokhtari, N., & Gheisari, M. (2021). Prolactin level in polycystic ovary syndrome (PCOS): An approach to the diagnosis and management. *Acta bio-medica: Atenei Parmensis, 92*(5), e2021291. https://doi.org/10.23750/abm.v92i5.9866
108. Moghadam, A. R. E., Moghadam, M. T., Hemadi, M., & Saki, G. (2022). Oocyte quality and aging. *JBRA Assisted Reproduction, 26*(1), 105.
109. Harris, I. D., Fronczak, C., Roth, L., & Meacham, R. B. (2011). Fertility and the aging male. *Reviews in Urology, 13*(4), e184–e190.
110. Fang, Y., Wang, Y., Peng, M., Xu, J., Fan, Z., Liu, C., Zhao, K., & Zhang, H. (2020). Effect of paternal age on offspring birth defects: a systematic review and meta-analysis. *Aging, 12*(24), 25373–25394. https://doi.org/10.18632/aging.104141
111. Brezina, P. R., Yunus, F. N., & Zhao, Y. (2012). Effects of pharmaceutical medications on male fertility. *Journal of Reproduction & Infertility, 13*(1), 3–11.
112. Pathak, M., Sharma, S., Kushwaha, P. P., & Kumar, S. (2020). Functional lead compounds and targets for the development of drugs for the treatment of male infertility. In *Phytochemicals as lead compounds for new drug discovery* (pp. 333–345). Elsevier.

113. Ghomeshi, A., Yang, B., & Masterson, T. A. (2023). The adverse effects of commonly used medications on male fertility: a comprehensive review. *F&S Reviews.*
114. Isojärvi, J. I., Löfgren, E., Juntunen, K. S., Pakarinen, A. J., Päivänsalo, M., Rautakorpi, I., & Tuomivaara, L. (2004). Effect of epilepsy and antiepileptic drugs on male reproductive health. *Neurology, 62*(2), 247–253. https://doi.org/10.1212/01.wnl.0000098936.46730.64
115. Evans-Hoeker, E. A., Eisenberg, E., Diamond, M. P., Legro, R. S., Alvero, R., Coutifaris, C., Casson, P. R., Christman, G. M., Hansen, K. R., Zhang, H., Santoro, N., Steiner, A. Z., & Network, R. M. (2018). Major depression, antidepressant use, and male and female fertility. *Fertility and Sterility, 109*(5), 879–887. https://doi.org/10.1016/j.fertnstert.2018.01.029
116. Fronczak, C. M., Kim, E. D., & Barqawi, A. B. (2012). The insults of illicit drug use on male fertility. *Journal of Andrology, 33*(4), 515–528. https://doi.org/10.2164/jandrol.110.011874
117. Rosati, L., Chianese, T., Mileo, A., De Falco, M., & Capaldo, A. (2023). Cocaine effects on reproductive behavior and fertility: An overview. *Veterinary Sciences, 10*(8), 484. https://doi.org/10.3390/vetsci10080484
118. Krzastek, S. C., Farhi, J., Gray, M., & Smith, R. P. (2020). Impact of environmental toxin exposure on male fertility potential. *Translational Andrology and Urology, 9*(6), 2797–2813. https://doi.org/10.21037/tau-20-685
119. Sansone, A., Di Dato, C., de Angelis, C., Menafra, D., Pozza, C., Pivonello, R., Isidori, A., & Gianfrilli, D. (2018). Smoke, alcohol and drug addiction and male fertility. *Reproductive Biology and Endocrinology: RB&E, 16*(1), 3. https://doi.org/10.1186/s12958-018-0320-7
120. Giviziez, C. R., Sanchez, E. G., Approbato, M. S., Maia, M. C., Fleury, E. A., & Sasaki, R. S. (2016). Obesity and anovulatory infertility: A review. *JBRA Assisted Reproduction, 20*(4), 240–245. https://doi.org/10.5935/1518-0557.20160046
121. Leisegang, K., Sengupta, P., Agarwal, A., & Henkel, R. (2021). Obesity and male infertility: Mechanisms and management. *Andrologia, 53*(1), Article e13617. https://doi.org/10.1111/and.13617
122. Wang, R., Qiang, Y., Gao, X., Yang, Q., & Li, B. (2022). Prevalence of non-communicable diseases and its association with tobacco smoking cessation intention among current smokers in Shanghai, China. *Tobacco Induced Diseases, 20*, 106. https://doi.org/10.18332/tid/155828
123. Harlev, A., Agarwal, A., Gunes, S. O., Shetty, A., & du Plessis, S. S. (2015). Smoking and male infertility: An evidence-based review. *The world Journal of Men's Health, 33*(3), 143–160. https://doi.org/10.5534/wjmh.2015.33.3.143
124. Kumar, S., Sharma, A., & Kshetrimayum, C. (2019). Environmental & occupational exposure & female reproductive dysfunction. *The Indian Journal of Medical Research, 150*(6), 532–545. https://doi.org/10.4103/ijmr.IJMR_1652_17
125. Marić, T., Fučić, A., & Aghayanian, A. (2021). Environmental and occupational exposures associated with male infertility. *Arhiv za higijenu rada i toksikologiju, 72*(3), 101–113. https://doi.org/10.2478/aiht-2021-72-3510
126. Rodprasert, W., Toppari, J., & Virtanen, H. E. (2023). Environmental toxicants and male fertility. *Best Practice & Research Clinical Obstetrics & Gynaecology, 86*, Article 102298.
127. Rooney, K. L., & Domar, A. D. (2018). The relationship between stress and infertility. *Dialogues in Clinical Neuroscience*, *20*(1), 41–47. https://doi.org/10.31887/DCNS.2018.20.1/klrooney
128. Matsas, A., Panopoulou, P., Antoniou, N., Bargiota, A., Gryparis, A., Vrachnis, N., Mastorakos, G., Kalantaridou, S. N., Panoskaltsis, T., Vlahos, N. F., & Valsamakis, G. (2023). Chronic stress in pregnancy is associated with low birth weight: A meta-analysis. *Journal of clinical medicine, 12*(24), 7686. https://doi.org/10.3390/jcm12247686
129. Yafi, F. A., Jenkins, L., Albersen, M., Corona, G., Isidori, A. M., Goldfarb, S., Maggi, M., Nelson, C. J., Parish, S., Salonia, A., Tan, R., Mulhall, J. P., & Hellstrom, W. J. (2016). Erectile dysfunction. *Nature Reviews. Disease Primers, 2*, 16003. https://doi.org/10.1038/nrdp.2016.3
130. Sadhir, S., & Pontzer, H. (2023). Impact of energy availability and physical activity on variation in fertility across human populations. *Journal of Physiological Anthropology, 42*(1), 1. https://doi.org/10.1186/s40101-023-00318-3

131. Orio, F., Muscogiuri, G., Ascione, A., Marciano, F., Volpe, A., La Sala, G., Savastano, S., Colao, A., & Palomba, S. (2013). Effects of physical exercise on the female reproductive system. *Minerva Endocrinologica, 38*(3), 305–319.
132. Osváth, P., Szűcs, M., Börzsei, D., Szabó, R., Lesi, Z. N., Turcsán, Z., Veszelka, M., Sebestyén, J., Juhász, B., Priksz, D., Varga, C., & Pósa, A. (2022). Andrological aspects of exercise: Moderate swimming protects against isoproterenol induced testis and semen abnormalities in rats. *Antioxidants (Basel, Switzerland), 11*(3), 436. https://doi.org/10.3390/antiox11030436
133. Qin, L., Yao, Z. Q., Chang, Q., Zhao, Y. L., Liu, N. N., Zhu, X. S., Liu, Q. Q., Wang, L. F., Yang, A. G., Gao, C. F., & Li, J. T. (2017). Swimming attenuates inflammation, oxidative stress, and apoptosis in a rat model of dextran sulfate sodium-induced chronic colitis. *Oncotarget, 8*(5), 7391–7404. https://doi.org/10.18632/oncotarget.14080

Chapter 3
AI Fundamentals

3.1 Introduction

AI is currently recognized as a specialized field within engineering, dedicated to addressing complex challenges through the implementation of innovative solutions. With ongoing advancements in electronic speed, capacity, and software programming, there is a foreseeable potential for computers to achieve a level of intelligence comparable to that of humans. Coined in 1956, the term "AI" encapsulates the science and engineering involved in creating intelligent machines, finding diverse applications in medical domains such as robotics, medical diagnosis, statistics, and human biology [1]. AI can be broadly divided into two branches: virtual and physical. The virtual branch employs informatics approaches, including deep learning, for tasks such as managing electronic health records and assisting physicians in making treatment decisions [2]. Machine learning, particularly deep learning, is a pivotal element in the virtual aspect of AI. It utilizes mathematical algorithms to enhance learning through experience, featuring three primary types: (1) supervised learning, which develops classification and prediction algorithms based on previous examples; (2) unsupervised learning, focusing on identifying patterns in data; and (3) reinforcement learning, which formulates strategies using sequences of rewards and punishments within a specific problem space. In contrast, the physical branch involves the development of robots designed to assist elderly patients, support surgeons, and utilize targeted nanorobots for innovative drug delivery systems [3]. In contrast, the physical aspect of AI encompasses the creation of robots intended to aid elderly patients, assist surgeons, and employ specialized nanorobots for advanced drug delivery systems [4]. Within the medical field, AI applications go beyond algorithms to involve physical entities like medical devices and advanced robots that actively participate in care delivery, commonly referred to as carebots. Notably, Japanese carebots showcase cutting-edge technology, functioning as assistant surgeons and even independently performing surgeries. However, ethical considerations pose a substantial challenge

KC. Santosh and D. G. Roy, *Artificial Intelligence for Human Fertility: Trends, Insights, and Predictions*, Studies in Computational Intelligence 1230,
https://doi.org/10.1007/978-981-95-1248-5_3

in this application, requiring meticulous standardization and comparative evaluation before considering widespread adoption. An emerging and promising application of AI in the medical field revolves around supervising the guided delivery of drugs using nanorobots. These minuscule robotic agents are meticulously crafted to address challenges linked to the diffusion of therapeutic agents into specific sites of interest. However, the seamless integration of these advanced AI applications into medical practices demands additional research, particularly in the realm of human–computer interactions. In the evaluation of humanoid robots, crucial factors such as their perceived humanity, the potential sense of eeriness they may elicit, and their overall attractiveness significantly shape how they are perceived in terms of acceptance, fear, or rejection [5].

AI-powered medical techniques are rapidly advancing and becoming practical solutions in clinical practice. Numerous studies have explored the diverse applications of AI in the medical field, revealing its potential across various areas. Examples include cardiovascular risk identification, early detection of atrial fibrillation, pulmonary function tests, glucose monitoring, clinical nephrology, seizure detection, as well as assessments of gait, posture, and tremors. Additionally, AI is proving beneficial in improving the intensive care unit environment and enhancing the efficiency of nursing and managerial activities in hospitals. The potential of AI extends to enhancing the prevention, detection, diagnosis, and treatment of diseases in healthcare [6]. Beyond clinical applications, AI is being integrated into medical practices for purposes such as digitizing medical records, conducting patient checkups using smart technologies, guiding surgeons during medication, treatment, and operations, and developing online platforms for patient appointments [7]. These applications have a transformative impact of AI in healthcare. Figure 3.1 depicts the broad spectrum of application areas where AI is making substantial advancements within the healthcare sector. It demonstrates the transformative impact of AI on various aspects of medical care. Below, a detailed description is provided for each segment to offer a comprehensive insight into its role in revolutionizing healthcare.

3.2 AI for Healthcare

Medical Image Diagnosis:

The advancement of automatic diagnosis capabilities and the development of diagnostic rules using medical image databases are continuously progressing. Numerous studies in the literature have concentrated on utilizing various types of images to predict complex and chronic diseases, with a primary focus on significant conditions such as cancer, Alzheimer's, cardiovascular disease, diabetic retinopathy, pulmonary diseases, neurological disorders, and others. These research endeavours aim to achieve precise disease diagnosis, segmentation phases, classification, object detection, identify distinctive features, and improve diagnostic accuracy, thereby enabling quicker and more accurate results for enhanced treatment planning. AI-based systems

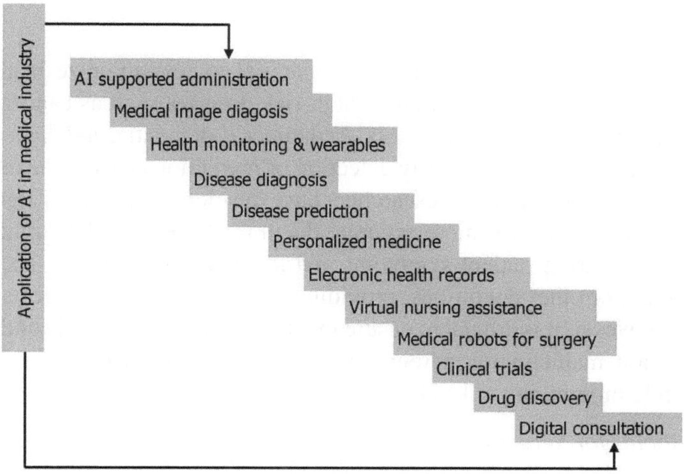

Fig. 3.1 Chart illustrating the applications of AI in the medical industry. The chart is structured as a descending staircase with each step representing a different application. Starting from the top: AI-supported administration, medical image diagnosis, health monitoring and wearables, disease diagnosis, disease prediction, personalized medicine, electronic health records, virtual nursing assistance, medical robots for surgery, clinical trials, drug discovery, and digital consultation. An arrow connects the last step back to the first, indicating a continuous cycle

across the board have showcased the integration of innovative computer-aided diagnosis architectures capable of diagnosing multiple diseases. The goal is to provide clinically meaningful endpoints, which are crucial for the seamless integration of AI into healthcare practice [8–11].

Digital Consultation:

Smart healthcare and online consultation have become increasingly popular and valuable initiatives within the healthcare system. These platforms offer patients a convenient and efficient online avenue for accessing medical advice and services. Traditional hospital visits can be costly and time-consuming, particularly in rural areas where healthcare access may be limited. Nowadays, people prioritize swift responses and continuous monitoring systems for their healthcare needs. In this digital age, telemedicine or digital consultation presents a mutually beneficial solution. A key aspect of digital consultation is the utilization of chatbots, which have emerged as the most popular tool in healthcare [12]. These chatbots function as digital medical guides, leveraging AI to accurately identify illnesses before a physician consultation. They assist both patients and doctors in disease search and provide comprehensive details about the detection process. AI-based healthcare applications play a vital role in guiding patients toward preventive measures and are likely to become integral components of future primary care services [13–15].

Disease Prediction:

Using AI for disease prediction has the potential to revolutionize healthcare by enabling the proactive identification of high-risk diseases such as cancer, COVID-19, cardiovascular disease, tuberculosis, Alzheimer's, dementia, and diabetes, which are often life-threatening [16]. Early detection or prediction can significantly reduce the risk of premature death. AI researchers have developed numerous algorithms to build intelligent models for more accurate diagnosis. These models utilize various approaches to analyze patient symptoms and identify abnormalities, such as fractures, tumours, or other conditions, providing quantitative measurements for faster diagnosis. However, it is crucial to ensure that these predictive models undergo thorough validation, maintain transparency, and are ethically deployed to maximize their benefits while minimizing risks [17].

Medical Robots for Surgery:

Robot-assisted medicine brings significant value to intervention quality and safety for both surgeons and patients. This technology spans various categories, including cost reduction, enhanced patient satisfaction, and improved clinical outcomes [18]. Procedures guided by robots involve the use of remotely controlled robotic systems, enabling surgeons to operate within the patient's body without extensive incisions. This approach enhances surgeon comfort and reduces exposure to ionizing radiation from the operating platform. However, the minimally invasive nature of soft robots' limits awareness of the operational workspace compared to open surgeries, where surgeons have full access to the surgical environment [19]. Exploring the historical, current, and future advancements in surgical assistance underscores the characteristics and advantages of medical robots, enabling high-precision movements and augmenting perception beyond human capabilities [20, 21].

Virtual Nursing Assistance:

Virtual nursing assistance involves providing nursing support and care remotely. This includes patient monitoring, medication management, wound care, and health education, facilitated through communication tools like video calls, phone calls, text messages, or secure messaging [22]. Additionally, it encompasses health risk assessment, decision support, personalized care planning based on the patient's needs and goals, remote patient engagement, such as medication and appointment reminders, and resource optimization to prevent hospital readmissions or emergency department visits. Moreover, AI plays a crucial role in augmenting nurses' capabilities, particularly during shortages of healthcare assistants [23].

Clinical Trials:

Clinical trials are pivotal in the discovery and introduction of new disease treatments to the market, as well as in advancing methods for disease detection, diagnosis, and prevention. The integration of AI into the design and execution phases of clinical trials offers significant benefits in terms of efficacy, safety, and cost containment [24]. Enhancing the early stages of trials has the potential to save time and resources, thereby promoting sustainability and efficient resource utilization. Furthermore, the adoption of digital innovation has the potential to revolutionize healthcare systems, leading to improved effectiveness and quality of care [25].

Health Monitoring and Wearables:

The rise of rapid aging and unexpected fatalities has spurred the demand for smart wearable systems, which play a crucial role in alleviating societal burdens [26]. These systems have become indispensable for adults, serving both as health monitors and personal assistants. With an array of smart wearable devices now available, individuals can promptly access vital health metrics such as heart rate, blood pressure, pulse, sleep patterns, neurological signals, movement disorders, mental well-being, metabolic rates, blood oxygen levels, pulmonary health, and environmental exposures [27]. This data facilitates continuous health assessment and enables timely intervention through precise treatment plans. By allowing health monitoring in the comfort of one's home, wearable systems reduce the need for physical checkups, cut down healthcare costs, and mitigate the risk of hospital admissions. Consequently, wearable systems have transformed healthcare and medicine by extending monitoring beyond clinical settings and enabling the anticipation of health events [28].

Electronic Health Records:

The digitalization of medical records worldwide has elevated EHRs to a pivotal position as a rich source of real-world data [29]. They complement traditional study methodologies by encompassing a diverse range of patient cases, thereby enhancing the generalizability of research findings. This is particularly significant for diseases that are rare and develop over extended periods. While much research has focused on core EHR functionalities like clinical support systems, computerized order entry systems, and health information exchange [30], numerous additional benefits have emerged. These include enhancements in clinical, organizational, and societal outcomes. Moreover, the continuous expansion of EHR systems underscores their effectiveness in modern healthcare delivery by streamlining administrative processes, fostering improved communication among healthcare providers, and bolstering the quality and safety of patient care [31].

AI-Supported Administration:

AI-supported administration utilizes artificial intelligence technologies to streamline administrative functions across diverse sectors. In healthcare, AI algorithms analyze vast datasets from electronic health records to optimize resource allocation, automate billing processes, and foster better communication between healthcare providers and patients [32]. Natural language processing algorithms aid in extracting valuable insights from unstructured data, while virtual assistants and chatbots provide continuous administrative assistance, enhancing accessibility and efficiency for both patients and healthcare professionals. Beyond healthcare, AI-supported administration extends to fields such as finance, education, and government, driving operational efficiency, facilitating informed decision-making, and enhancing service delivery across various industries [33].

Personalized Medicine:

In recent years, personalized medicine has sparked significant interest, stemming from the recognition that individuals possess distinct and multifaceted traits at molecular, physiological, environmental exposure, and behavioural levels [34]. As a result, there is a belief that customizing interventions for diseases based on these unique characteristics can improve effectiveness. This endeavour toward true personalized medicine entails evaluating eight essential elements: access to healthcare, genetics and genomics, tissue biomarkers, imaging and radiology, environmental exposure, wireless monitoring, behaviours and personality, and epigenetic modifications. Additionally, domains such as disease prevention, intensive health monitoring, digital therapeutics, and interventions concerning fertility and sterility play pivotal roles in this paradigm [30]. The implementation of these innovative approaches is supported by educating and training healthcare professionals, leading to improved efficiency and cost-effectiveness. This approach shows promise in understanding individual patient responses to interventions and tailoring treatments accordingly [35].

Disease Diagnosis:

In recent years, nations worldwide have grappled with numerous human health challenges that strain healthcare delivery. Despite significant strides in medical diagnostics to detect and treat chronic diseases, obstacles like high diagnostic costs, infrastructure shortages, equipment deficits, and a lack of skilled technicians persist, limiting patient access to care [36]. Human error further complicates accurate diagnostics, given the complexity of interpreting medical information. The integration of AI offers promising prospects for enhancing diagnostic accuracy and efficiency. Certain forms of AI, like machine learning and deep learning, enable the effective examination of extensive datasets, identifying patterns, and deriving critical insights. This facilitates predictions for medical diagnoses and personalized treatment recommendations [37]. Timely and accurate disease diagnosis is pivotal for effective treatment planning and patient well-being on a day-to-day basis [16].

Drug Discovery:

Drug discovery is indeed a complex and time-consuming process that requires a multidisciplinary approach. Despite advancements in understanding biological systems, the quest for new drug molecules remains challenging and expensive [38]. Modern drug discovery pipelines involve various stages, including target identification and validation, lead candidate screening, and optimization for desired properties like affinity and metabolic stability. The integration of AI and ML, together with big data, offers significant opportunities in drug discovery. These technologies streamline tasks such as predicting protein folding, virtual screening, designing new drugs, and repurposing existing ones. Moreover, AI has revolutionized drug discovery and is poised to become an essential tool for identifying novel drugs and targets in the pharmaceutical sector [39–41].

3.3 Methods

Introducing a new AI system involves several pivotal stages, including acquiring datasets, ensuring data integrity, enhancing computational power, refining algorithms, optimizing cost efficiency, establishing laboratory settings, assessing the importance of features and instances, defining target labels and desired outcomes, and understanding relevant constraints. Consequently, effectively integrating a predictive model into clinical decision-making demands meticulous consideration of these diverse factors [42]. Figure 3.2 illustrates the different stages of AI model implementation.

Availability of Datasets:

Data plays a crucial role in developing AI models, yet its availability in reproductive medicine remains limited. AI models typically perform best when trained on large datasets, so the constraints of small sample sizes can hinder their effectiveness. However, technological advancements have improved access to data in recent years. Various platforms, including EHR, publicly accessible datasets (such as those

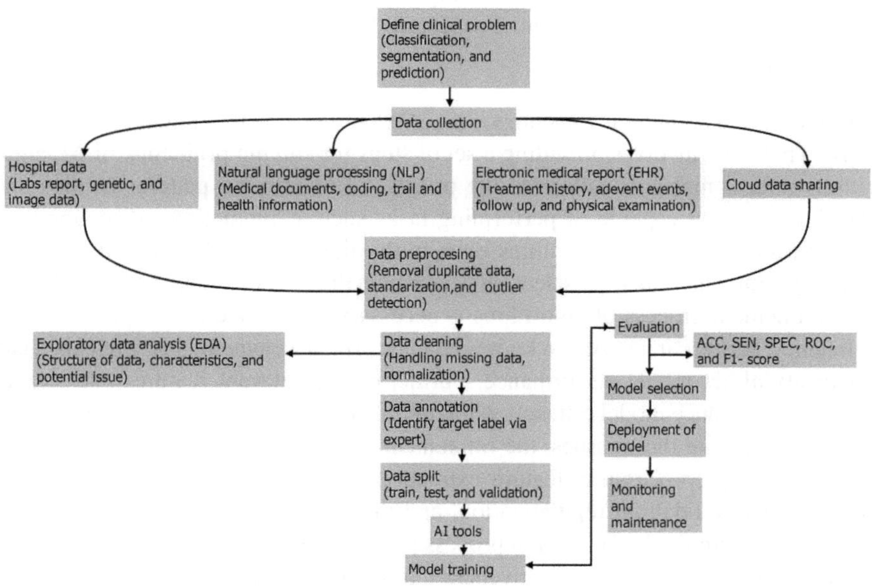

Fig. 3.2 Chart illustrating a clinical data processing workflow. It begins with defining a clinical problem, followed by data collection from hospital data, natural language processing (NLP), and electronic medical reports (EHR). Data is shared via cloud and undergoes preprocessing to remove duplicates and detect outliers. Exploratory data analysis (EDA) examines data structure and potential issues. Data cleaning addresses missing data and normalization, followed by annotation and splitting into train, test, and validation sets. AI tools are used for model training. Evaluation metrics include ACC, SEN, SPEC, ROC, and F1-score. The process concludes with model selection, deployment, and ongoing monitoring and maintenance

provided by NIH, CDC, and WHO), research collaborations involving clinical trials and observational studies, as well as contributions from medical journals and data marketplaces like Kaggle, PhysioNet, and MIMIC-II, have expanded the availability of medical data. It is imperative for researchers utilizing these datasets to adhere to ethical guidelines, comply with data privacy regulations, and obtain appropriate institutional review board approvals, particularly when dealing with sensitive patient information, such as reproductive health data [43–45].

Advancing Computer Power:

AI systems deal with distinct types of datasets, sometimes massive, containing millions or billions of parameters. Training these models requires extensive computational resources to process the data and adjust the parameters to minimize errors. Fast processing speed and low latency are two fundamental requirements during real-time processing. Additionally, optimization and tuning provide an efficient and improved AI model, with numerous iterations running, which can be computationally intensive. Lastly, advanced infrastructure allows AI systems to scale up to handle larger workloads, and AI algorithms often involve complex mathematical operations that demand high computational resources. Moreover, achieving accurate results in real-time and tackling increasingly complex problems requires the upliftment of computational power as an essential aspect of the AI domain [46, 47].

Refining Algorithms:

Algorithms are a fundamental component of AI systems; without them, AI wouldn't exist. Their role involves providing a set of steps for solving problems. In AI, algorithms offer a means to automate the process of identifying patterns in data and develop a system capable of performing tasks such as predictions, detection, and classification. Plenty of algorithms exist in the literature, each based on different learning strategies, and their selection depends on the target variable and class labels. The refinement process of algorithms is necessary to upgrade model performance, efficiency, and accuracy. As we know, data is a primary element, and noisy data can adversely affect model performance. Furthermore, irrelevant features and similar features can reduce model efficacy, while imbalanced data can lead to biased predictions. To mitigate these issues, the refinement of algorithms includes several steps such as data preprocessing, feature extraction, feature reduction, hyperparameter tuning, cross-validation, regularization, and the continuous selection of advanced algorithms, refining the evaluation process [48]. By following these steps, improvements in performance and effectiveness can be achieved, ultimately fulfilling the goal of an AI system.

Optimizing Cost-Effectiveness:

AI systems, developed across various domains, including healthcare, bring forth significant benefits. In healthcare settings, AI functions as a tool for computer-aided diagnoses, assisting clinicians in crafting effective treatment strategies. The optimization of costs is pivotal in healthcare, sometimes resulting in reduced interest among individuals in disease diagnosis. Consequently, many suffer globally from untreated conditions. AI-assisted models excel in identifying high-risk conditions through a range of diverse features. In reality, numerous diseases significantly contribute to mortality, morbidity, and disability. Automated AI models span a broad spectrum, from detecting breast cancer, Covid-19, TB, and diabetes to addressing fertility issues (sperm selection and semen analysis), evaluation and selection of oocytes, embryo selection, PCOS, Alzheimer's dementia, and analyzing liver fat, sarcopenia, and osteoporosis, and many more [49]. Furthermore, AI facilitates automated cardiovascular risk assessment and aids in detecting transmitted diseases. Overall, the integration of AI revolutionizes healthcare, particularly benefiting regions with limited and costly medical resources [50].

Establishing Laboratory Setup:

Many factors warrant careful consideration when integrating a new system into the laboratory, necessitating thorough evaluation before reaching a decision. Introducing an AI system requires attention to various elements [51]:

User Interface:

The visual display on the screen should indicate the state of the user interface for better understanding and navigation. Scalability: The system should have high scalability to meet the laboratory's needs, considering factors such as data volume, user numbers, and integration with existing workflows and protocols.

Training:

Adequate training for users is essential, with information provided by the manufacturer to ensure proficiency in system usage. Support: Technical support should be available in case of failures, with clear communication at response times. Follow-up: Continuous learning is crucial, with algorithms regularly updated to accommodate new data. Maintenance and Monitoring: The manufacturer should provide information on maintenance and monitoring plans to ensure the system's ongoing accuracy and impartiality.

Cost:

Cost considerations should align with the laboratory's budget and investment capacity. Ethics: Ethical considerations are paramount, evaluating the system's impact on patient care and outcomes to ensure it operates ethically and avoids harm or negative impacts on patients. Confidentiality and security measures for patient data should meet standards like ISO 27002-2021 and IEC 62304. Transparency: Transparent models enhance clinical decision-making, while opaque "black-box" systems can lead to uncertainty about treatment success responsibility. It's crucial to understand the risks, side effects, benefits, and confidence levels of each clinical decision before delegating decision-making to machines. Opaque models may introduce biases and increase the risk of imbalanced outcomes.

Data:

Data quality encompasses various aspects such as accuracy, completeness, timeliness, relevance, consistency, and reliability. Access to high-quality data is crucial for an AI system to deliver accurate and reliable results. The future failure of AI systems can be attributed to unreliable and non-generalizable data during model building. Certain models are based on specific populations, and if data across populations lack homogeneity, the model's accuracy may be compromised. Performance: It refers to how effectively and efficiently an AI system achieves its intended goals, including factors such as accuracy, speed, and reliability. Evaluating the system's performance entails measuring it against relevant metrics and benchmarks to ensure it meets the desired standards.

Features and Instances Importance:

Input data typically comprises a set of input features or variables. When an AI model generates a prediction, it leans more heavily on certain features over others. Consequently, some features hold greater importance for the model, while others are less influential. Hence, the accuracy of the model's prediction is directly linked to the quality of its features. This determines the extent to which each feature contributes to the model's prediction, thereby gauging the utility of specific variables for the given model and prediction. Overall, the significance of each feature is assessed using numerical values, with higher and lower scores denoting the top and bottom features, respectively. Furthermore, the interrelationship among features, encompassing input and target labels, can be readily discerned. By scrutinizing variable importance, irrelevant features can be pinpointed and easily excluded. Trimming the number of non-meaningful features can hasten model processing or even enhance its performance. Common methods for evaluating feature importance include correlation analysis, permutation testing, single-variable prediction, and model-dependent feature importance techniques like linear regression, logistic regression, decision trees, and neural networks [52–55]. Moreover, the quantity of instances significantly influences prediction outcomes. An instance denotes a single data point or example from a dataset. If instance numbers are low, there's a possibility of encountering underfitting issues (high bias and low variance), rendering the model more susceptible to data outliers or noise, potentially leading to less accurate predictions. Conversely, if the dataset is large or unrefined, containing noise, the model might exhibit high variance with low bias, resulting in overfitting. In either scenario, the model fails to yield accurate results. Various strategies, such as noise reduction, enhancing model complexity, prolonging training duration, augmenting training data, employing cross-validation techniques, and adopting ensemble methods, are employed to mitigate these issues and develop a well-fitted model. Additionally, both feature and instance importance are pivotal concepts influencing model performance [56].

Specifying Desired Result and Target Label:

In AI model design, the target labels and desired outcomes are closely intertwined. The target represents the ultimate output that the AI model aims to provide, whether it's categorical or continuous. On the other hand, the label reflects the true outcome of the target and is assigned to the training dataset. Following training, the AI model is then tasked with processing unlabelled data for prediction. Within healthcare, labels are pivotal in classification tasks, where outputs are categorical, such as in disease diagnosis [56, 57]. Meanwhile, regression tasks deal with continuous values, like heart rate or brain activity monitoring, and vital sign tracking for clinical applications. In regression, the outcome always comes in terms of value, and that value indicates the next label of patient's health condition [58]. Therefore, both classification and regression models offer significant benefits, potentially reshaping the clinical landscape.

Understanding Limitations:

AI research in healthcare is accelerating rapidly, with the potential application being demonstrated across various domains of medicine, and reproductive medicine is not exceptional. However, there are currently limited examples of such techniques being successfully deployed into clinical practice. Different types of downsides are still present in AI applications, which can restrict us from exploring AI widely. The key challenges are data privacy and security, high implementation cost, limited data size, and lack of transparency. The top five key reasons to interpret reproduction AI studies with caution [59]. There are no generalizability assessment, an unbalanced dataset, a small sample size, limited performance metrics reported, and lack of a universal understanding of inner workings. Firstly, an AI-based algorithm should be tested for generalizability across clinics and using a wide spectrum of sample types available in clinical practice. However, some of the studies presented here describe AI-based algorithms trained using data from a single clinic or with very specific inclusion criteria limiting their clinical applicability in other conditions. Secondly, an AI algorithm is trained to find the best performance with the specific data presented to it. When the training set is highly unbalanced, the model may be prone to intrinsic bias; thus, the description of the algorithm should include the actions taken to avoid such bias.

Limited dataset size may result in overfitting, compromising the model's ability to generalize. Common metrics used to evaluate AI model performance include accuracy and the area under the curve, and receiver operating characteristic curve. However, with these metrics alone, a reader cannot perform a deeper performance analysis while dealing with biological parameters, for example, if the model is more prone to error in one class or the other [60]. Good practice in this area is to be fully transparent by reporting the confusion matrix or presenting a table with the testing case, prediction, and true results. In recent days, AI models have mostly been a black box, and this opacity has ethical and legal risks and liability issues, which may lead to distrust of patients and clinicians of AI [61]. Moreover, the application of AI in reproductive medicine becomes beneficial when researchers understand these five key challenges and limitations [62].

3.4 Feature Handling

Developing a robust AI model that performs well on unseen data depends heavily on identifying informative features within the dataset. The process of building a predictive AI model typically begins with dataset preprocessing, which includes quality control and dimensionality reduction. This step is essential for producing a high-quality dataset that reduces computational complexity and enhances learning performance. When faced with a large number of input features, dimensionality reduction becomes critical. It generally falls into two categories: feature selection and feature extraction. Feature selection involves choosing a subset of the original features, while feature extraction transforms the original features into a new set of composite features. Each method has its strengths and limitations. Feature extraction can improve discriminative power and support data visualization but may lack interpretability. Conversely, feature selection retains meaningful, interpretable features, making it particularly valuable in domains like medicine, even if it sometimes compromises accuracy [63, 64]. Given our focus on medical applications, we emphasize feature selection. These methods can be classified into two types based on their evaluation strategy: individual evaluation (or feature ranking), where features are assessed independently and assigned relevance scores, and subset evaluation, where combinations of features are evaluated to identify the most effective subset.

3.4.1 Feature Selection

Feature selection techniques are categorized into three main methods: filters, embedded, and wrappers, based on their interaction with learning methods. Table 3.1 outlines the benefits and drawbacks of each selection method along with examples.

Filter Methods:

Filter methods are the simplest and most efficient feature selection techniques, operating independently of any learning algorithm [65]. They evaluate features based on intrinsic data characteristics such as correlation with the target variable or variance, making them fast, scalable, and generalizable. These methods are broadly categorized as univariate, which assesses each feature individually, and multivariate, which evaluate feature subsets simultaneously [66, 67]. While univariate filters are favoured for high-dimensional datasets due to their speed and simplicity, they fail to detect redundancy or feature interactions, which may hinder model performance. Multivariate filters address these issues by considering feature interdependencies, but they are computationally more demanding and, like univariate filters, do not account for interactions with the learning algorithm.

Table 3.1 Benefits and drawbacks of three feature selection methods

Methods	Benefits	Drawbacks	Examples
Filter univariate	Fast and scalable, Independent of classifier, and reduced risk of overfitting	Feature dependencies are not modelled, and Interaction with the classifier is not modelled	Chi-squared test, Fisher's exact test, Pearson correlation, Information Gain, t-test, Mann–Whitney U test
Filter-multivariate	Can model feature dependencies, independent of the classifier, and less risk of overfitting	Slower and not as scalable as univariate filters, Interaction with the classifier is not modelled	Fast-correlation-based filter, minimal redundancy, maximum relevance, and relief-based algorithms
Wrapper	Model feature dependencies, better performance than filter method, and model interaction with classifier	Slower than filter and embedded methods, and more prone to overfitting, selected features are classifier dependent	Sequential forward and backward selection, randomized hill climbing, genetic algorithm, recursive feature elimination
Embedded	Model feature dependencies, faster than wrapper method, and model interaction with classifier	Slower than filter methods, selected features are classifier dependent	Random forest, lasso, or elastic net regression

Wrapper Methods:

Wrapper methods incorporate a learning algorithm into the feature selection process, evaluating feature subsets based on the classifier's performance [68]. Search strategies such as forward selection, backward elimination, or recursive feature elimination are used to explore the feature space and identify optimal subsets. Although wrappers tend to produce higher accuracy than filters by considering feature interactions with the classifier, they are computationally intensive and classifier dependent. This dependence means the selected subset may not generalize across different models, increasing the risk of overfitting [69]. Additionally, wrappers output a single "best" feature subset rather than a ranked list, which eliminates the need to set selection thresholds but makes individual feature importance less interpretable.

Embedded Methods:

Embedded methods integrate feature selection into the model training process, allowing the classifier to determine feature importance by adjusting internal parameters [70]. This is typically achieved by modifying the objective function or adding a regularization term to penalize less relevant features. Embedded methods offer a balance between filter and wrapper approaches by combining classifier interaction with relatively low computational cost. Although more demanding than filter methods, they are more efficient than wrappers and often yield better generalization performance due to their ability to incorporate classifier bias during feature selection [71]. Common examples include decision trees, LASSO regression, and other regularized models.

In medical applications, while filters are commonly favoured for feature selection, the increasing array of available techniques presents a challenge in selecting the optimal method for a given problem. The "no free lunch theorem" highlights that no single algorithm can universally excel across all problem sets. This holds true for feature selection methods, each with its own distinct advantages and disadvantages (see Table 3.1), relying on specific metrics and underlying assumptions. Numerous researchers have conducted comparative analyses, assessing the performance of various feature selection methods across predictive models. These studies consistently stress that there is no universally superior method; rather, the choice depends on the specific dataset under analysis and the objectives researchers aim to achieve. According to the literature, several methods are frequently utilized, such as CFS [72], consistency-based filter [73], interact [74], information gain [75], reliefF [76], and recursive feature elimination for support vector machine [77]. Table 3.2 outlines the characteristics of each method to support a clearer understanding of their strategic approaches, whereas Table 3.3 provides practical recommendations tailored to different problem contexts [71].

Additionally, aside from these three traditional methods, other approaches such as hybrid, integrative, and ensemble feature selection methods are widely utilized in various applications [78–80]. Hybrid methods streamline the feature search space by integrating the filter step, thus enabling the subsequent use of computationally intensive wrapper or embedded methods for high-dimensional datasets [81]. Integrative approaches leverage external information to refine the feature search space before the reduced feature set undergoes a wrapper or embedded method to produce the final feature subset [82]. In ensemble methods, multiple feature selection techniques' outputs are amalgamated to obtain the ultimate set of selected features [83]. Many documented case studies underscore the practical effectiveness of feature selection techniques across various domains like medical imaging [84], biomedical signal processing [85], and the analysis of DNA microarray and SNP data [16]. Although hybrid methods are seen as advanced due to their resource dependencies, traditional approaches still offer satisfactory outcomes in real-time medical applications.

3.4.2 Feature Extraction

Feature extraction methods are essential in healthcare analytics, serving as a bridge between raw medical data and actionable insights. These techniques enable the conversion of complex and high-dimensional data into a structured form that is easier to interpret and analyze. Their role is particularly crucial in uncovering clinically meaningful patterns that may not be immediately evident in the unprocessed data. Given the diversity of medical data—ranging from images and physiological signals to genetic information and clinical text—a wide array of tools and techniques

Table 3.2 Methods and their description

Methods	Description
CFS	This method is a multivariate filtering technique that picks feature subsets uncorrelated with each other yet demonstrating notable correlation with the class
Consistency-based filter	It is a multivariate technique that additionally selects feature subsets based on their consistency with the class and then employs an inconsistency criterion to determine an acceptable rate of data reduction
Interact	The algorithm functions in two stages: initially, it calculates the symmetrical uncertainty of all features, arranging them accordingly. Subsequently, it assesses each variable individually based on its consistency contribution, selecting only those whose consistency contribution exceeds a predetermined threshold
Information gain	It is a basic univariate filter that calculates the mutual information for each attribute and class, generating an ordered ranking of all features
Relief	This popular multivariate filter, an extension of the previous Relief version, utilizes nearest neighbours. It randomly selects samples and identifies nearest neighbours from the same class, excluding all others. Comparing the values of the selected sample with the hits and misses, it updates the relevance score for each feature. A valuable feature is anticipated to have values resembling those of examples from the same class and differing from examples from other classes
Recursive feature elimination for support vector machine	It is an embedded method where, during an iterative process of training an SVM classifier, features are selected, and the least important ones are eliminated based on the weights in the SVM solution

has been developed and extensively documented in the literature to address various analytical needs. The core goal of feature extraction is to reduce the dimensionality of the input data while retaining the most informative components. This often involves transforming the original variables into a new set of features, either through linear or nonlinear combinations. These derived features usually differ in form and scale from the original variables but encapsulate the same, or even more relevant, information. Contrary to the belief that reducing the number of features might lead to underfitting, feature extraction typically enhances model performance by eliminating redundant or noisy data, which is common in healthcare datasets.

Over the years, extensive research has led to the development of specialized feature extraction techniques tailored to different data types. In medical imaging, features such as shape, texture, and intensity are commonly extracted. These approaches aim to distill complex datasets into features that can improve the accuracy, interpretability, and efficiency of predictive models. Recognizing the significance of feature extraction, researchers have continually refined these methods to support

Table 3.3 Recommendations for specific feature selection approaches customized to different scenarios [84]

Approaches	Correlation	Non	Input	Target	No. features >>
	Redundancy	Linearity	Noise	Noise	No. samples
CFS	*	*	*	***	****
Consistency	*	*	*	***	**
Interact	*	*	*	***	***
Info-gain	*	*	*	***	***
ReliefF	****	*****	*****	*****	**
mRMR	****	***	*****	**	*
SVM-REF (Linear kernel)	****	*	*	****	*****
SVM-REF (Nonlinear kernel)	****	*****	***	****	–
Wrapper SVM	*	*	***	****	**
Wrapper C4.5	**	***	***	***	***

applications such as diagnosis, prognosis, and treatment planning [86]. The literature is rich with methodologies that emphasize both theoretical soundness and practical utility. Tables 3.4 and 3.5 summarize key feature extraction techniques, presenting their conceptual underpinnings and highlighting their relevance in various clinical contexts.

3.4.3 Data Balancing

Specifically in public healthcare, class imbalance is a pervasive issue that can significantly degrade the performance and clinical utility of machine learning models, especially when predicting rare outcomes such as early-stage cancers, adverse drug reactions, or successful treatment responses. To address this, a variety of data balancing techniques have been adopted [87]. Oversampling methods such as the SMOTE and ADASYN generate synthetic examples of the minority class to improve model sensitivity without simply duplicating existing data. These have been widely applied in medical domains including cancer diagnosis, sepsis detection, and reproductive outcome prediction. Conversely, undersampling methods like random undersampling, Tomek links, and ENN reduce the majority class to prevent bias, although they risk discarding clinically relevant data. Hybrid methods, such as SMOTE combined with Tomek links or ENN, offer a balanced trade-off between class representation and data quality. Additionally, algorithmic approaches such as cost-sensitive learning and class weighting are integrated into model training to penalize misclassification of the minority class, enhancing fairness and robustness without altering the dataset. In medical imaging, data augmentation and the use of GANs have also

Table 3.4 Conceptual view of Linear-FE methods

Concept framework	Methods				
	PCA	LDA	ICA	SVD	**NMF**
Objective	Enhance variance	Increase class disaffiliation	Increase statistical independence	Enhance reconstruction error	Extract hidden pattern
Operation	Unsupervised	Supervised	Unsupervised	Unsupervised	Unsupervised
Data characteristics	Handle skewed data	Perform better with uniformly distributed data	Handle higher-order statistics	Handle spare and nonlinear data	Naturally represents an additive combination
Iteration	No	No	Yes	Yes	Yes
Topology	Random projection	Random projection	Random projection	Random projection	Random projection
Computational speed	Medium	High	Very low speed	Very low speed	Low speed
Scalability	Low scalability	High scalability	Low scalability	High scalability	Low scalability
Tuning of parameters	No. of components	None	No. of components and iterations	No. of components and iterations	No. of features and iterations
Computational complexity	$O\left(d^2n+n^3\right)$	$O\left(d^2n\right), n>d;$ $O\left(d^3\right), d>n$	$O(2di(d+1)+n]$	$O\left(d^2n+n^3\right)$	$O(t\left(mnr+mr^2+nr^2\right)$
Weakness	Limited to a linear projection	Suffer from class singularity issue	Require high training time	Not suitable for nonlinear data	Convergence issues
Transformation	Eigen decomposition	Class discrimination by scatter matrices	Non-Gaussian distribution	SVD theorem	Decomposition of multivariate data

Table 3.5 Conceptual comparison of nonlinear FE

Concept framework	Methods				
	NCA	KPCA	Autoencoder	T-sne	Isomap
Objective	Improves nearest neighbour classification	Linearly separate data	To minimize the difference between the input data and the reconstructed data	Preserve local structure	Preserve geodesic pairwise distance
Operation	Supervised	Unsupervised	Unsupervised	Unsupervised	Unsupervised
Data characteristics	Perform better with nonlinear and overlapping data set,	Perform better with nonlinear data	Perform time-series, or image data	Perform better with numeric data	Handle spare and noisy data
Iteration	Yes	No	Yes	Yes	No
Topology	Manifold	Manifold	Manifold	Manifold	Manifold
Computational speed	Medium	Fast	Faster	Medium	Medium
Scalability	Medium	High	Low	Medium	Medium
Tunning parameter	No. of components	No. of components, kernel	No. of layers	No. of components and iteration	No. of components and nearest neighbours
Computational complexity	$O(n^2 dm)$	$O(n^3)$	$O\left(\sum_{i=1}^{L} n_1 \cdot m_i + \sum_{j=1}^{L'} p_j \cdot q_j\right)$	$O(n^2)$	$O[d \log(c) n \log(n)] + O[n^2(c + \log(n)] + O(kn^2)$
Weakness	Risk of overfitting	Required high training time	Prone to overfitting	Provide only 2 or 3 features	Suffer from tropical instability
Transformation	Linear mapping	Kernel mapping	Encoding and decoding	Conditional probabilities	Neighbourhood graph, geodesic distance

(continued)

Table 3.5 (continued)

Concept framework	Methods			
	Umap	LLE	**LE**	**MDS**
Objective	Preserve the global structure and local relationships of data points	Preserve local properties	Preserve local distances	Preserve Euclidean pairwise distances
Operation	Unsupervised	Unsupervised	Unsupervised	Unsupervised
Data characteristics	Handle spare and nonlinear data	Handle spare and nonlinear data	Handle noisy data	Perform better with relational data
Iteration	Yes	Yes	No	Yes
Topology	Manifold	Manifold	Manifold	Manifold
Computational speed	Faster	Faster	Faster	Faster
Scalability	Very high	Less	More	More
Tunning parameter	No. of nearest neighbours and iterations	No. of components, iterations and nearest neighbour	No. of components and nearest neighbours	No. of component and iterations
Computational complexity	$O(n\log(n)\cdot d+t\cdot n\cdot k)$	$O\left(d\ \log(c)n\log(n)\right)+O\left(dnc^3\right)+O\left(kn^2\right)$	$O\left(d\ \log(c)n\log(n)\right)+O\left(dnc^3\right)+O\left(kn^2\right)$	$O\left(n^3\right)$
Weakness	Performance affected due to high dimensional spare data	Consume memory	May produce disconnected neighbourhood graph	Require high computation and memory to calculate dissimilarity matrix
Transformation	Initial embedding	Neighbourhood graph, reconstruction weights	Neighbourhood graph, weight update of edges	Dissimilarity matrix via Euclidean distance

emerged as powerful techniques for balancing datasets by synthesizing realistic yet rare clinical patterns. Collectively, these approaches play a vital role in improving the performance, generalizability, and clinical acceptance of AI systems in healthcare [88].

3.5 AI Tools

AI tools are rapidly emerging as a transformative force in computer science, with the potential to revolutionize medical practice and healthcare delivery. This section delves into recent advancements in medical science, highlighting the wide array of AI approaches being employed. The literature offers a comprehensive overview of AI tools, providing a roadmap for the development of effective, reliable, and safe AI systems. These tools enable the creation of intelligent machines that mimic human cognitive functions, such as learning and problem-solving, using algorithms or rule-based systems. AI is not a single, uniform technology; rather, it encompasses various subfields that, either individually or in combination, enhance applications with intelligence. Different sets of rules or algorithms have been crafted to allow computer programs to autonomously improve through experience. Among the most prominent clinical applications are those in cardiovascular health, dermatology, obstetrics and gynaecology, neurology, infectious diseases, oncology, and more. Within these fields, key application areas focus on diagnosis and treatment recommendations.

In this context, the most employed algorithms include (1) Support Vector Machine (SVM), (2) Decision Tree (DT), (3) Random Decision Forest (RDF), (4) Naïve Bayes (NB), (5) Logistic Regression (LR), (6) K-Nearest Neighbour (K-NN), (7) Mulit-Layer Perceptron (MLP), and (8) Artificial Neural Network (ANN), which are regarded as conventional approaches. Extensive research has further demonstrated that ensemble methods like bagging, boosting, and stacking are widely recognized for their ability to enhance the performance of individual algorithms across various applications. Prominent ensemble classifiers, such as (1) AdaBoost (ADA), (2) Gradient Boosting Machine (GBM), (3) Extreme Gradient Boosting (XGB) and (4) Categorical Boosting (CBT), and (5) Light Gradient Boosting Machine (LGBM) are frequently used in medical science applications, including fertility treatments.

Conventional Tools:

These tools are fundamental or refer to traditional methods that are widely used and established in the field of AI over time. It is well understood and often serves as a starting point for more complex or modern AI systems. The description of the tools is given below:

SVM:

This algorithm was invented by Cortes and Vapnik [89], and the fundamental idea is to create a hyperplane that separates the input data for class 1 or class -1. The large scale of classification problems is solvable using SVM. Assume $\{(X_i, Y_i) : i \in [m]\}$

with $[m] = \{1, 2, \ldots, m\}$ be a set of training examples, where $X_i \in \mathbb{R}^n$ indicates the input data and $Y_i \in \{-1, 1\}$ stands for the corresponding label. The key objective of SVM is to learn a hyperplane $\langle W, X \rangle + b = 0$ with $b \in \mathbb{R}$ and $W \in \mathbb{R}^n$ to be estimated by using given set of training examples. To learn the maximal $W \in \mathbb{R}^n$ and $b \in \mathbb{R}$, we consider the two scenarios: linearly separable and inseparable training datasets.

Scenario 1: linearly separable training datasets: the maximum $W \in \mathbb{R}^n$ and $b \in \mathbb{R}$ can be obtained by handling the following convex hard margin SVM model $\min_{W\in\mathbb{R}^n, b\in\mathbb{R}} \frac{1}{2}\|w\|^2 \text{s.t. } y_i(\langle W, X\rangle + b) \geq 1, i \in [m]$, where $\|\cdot\|$ represents the Euclidean norm and $\langle , \rangle$ represents the inner product. The constraints of the hard margin SVM require correct classifications of all training samples.

Scenario 2: For linearly inseparable training datasets, the popular technique is to allow violations of the constraints of (1) and then penalize these violations in the objective function, which allows us to yield the following unconstrainted soft - margin SVM model $\min_{W\in\mathbb{R}^n, b\in\mathbb{R}} \frac{1}{2}\|W\|^2 + \beta \sum_{i=1}^{m} \ell(u_i)$ where $\beta > 0$ indicates the penalty parameters and $\ell(\cdot)$ stands for the soft margin loss function, and for any $i = 1, \ldots, m$, $u_i = 1 - y_i(\langle W, X\rangle + b) \in \mathbb{R}$. The soft margin loss function and it has been widely studied and applied in many fields such as image classification, ML, disease diagnosis, and so on [90–92]. The soft margin SVM is currently being developed and is encountering numerous challenges when solving large-scale classification.

DT:

The DT method is a powerful statistical tool used for classification, prediction, interpretation, and data manipulation, with several potential applications in medical research [93]. The basic structure of a DT relies on nodes and branches, which are its primary components. To build a model, three main steps are involved: splitting, stopping, and pruning. In a simple DT model, a binary target variable Y (0 or 1) and two continuous variables, $X1$ and $X2$, each ranging from 0 to 1, are considered. There are three types of nodes in a DT: the root node, internal nodes, and leaf nodes. The root node represents the initial decision point and subdivides all records into two or more mutually exclusive subsets. Internal nodes, also called chance nodes, represent the possible choices available at each point in the tree structure. The top edge of an internal node connects it to its parent node, while the bottom edge connects it to its child nodes or leaf nodes. The leaf node represents the result based on a combination of decisions or events. Branches in the model represent paths from the root node, through the internal nodes, to the leaf nodes, with each path signifying a classification decision rule based on "if–then" logic.

During the splitting phase, only input variables related to the target variable are used to split parent nodes into purer child nodes. The process starts by identifying the most important input variable for splitting, then dividing the records at the root node and subsequent internal nodes into two or more categories (or bins) based on the variable's status. This continues until a predetermined homogeneity or stopping criterion is met. These criteria include entropy, Gini index, classification error, information gain, gain ratio, and the towing rule [92]. The stopping rule is applied when the model becomes too complex or risks being overly fitted to the existing data, leading to very few records in each leaf. To avoid these problems, common parameters are used, such as: (a) the minimum number of records in a leaf; (b) the minimum number of records in a node before splitting; and (c) the depth (i.e., the number of steps) from the root node to any leaf. Finally, pruning is applied when the tree becomes overly complex. In this process, a large DT is built first, then pruned to an optimal size by reducing nodes that contain less information. Common techniques include creating subtrees by considering error prediction proportions, cross-validation, chi-square tests, and multiple-comparison adjustment methods [94].

RDF:

RDF is a decision tree-based method widely used for both classification and regression tasks. It constructs an ensemble of hundreds of decision trees with randomized inputs and splits, helping to mitigate the biggest drawback of a single decision tree—overfitting. In Random Forest, overfitting is addressed by averaging the predictions of individual trees and comparing them to the actual output. The Random Forest classifier operates using bagging, also known as bootstrap aggregation. This process begins by selecting random subsets of data from the entire dataset, known as bootstrap samples, to create individual models. Each model is trained independently, with row sampling done with replacement (bootstrapping), and each produces its own result. The final prediction is made by combining the results from all models through majority voting, where the most frequently predicted outcome is selected. It is important to note that the majority voting process varies depending on the task. For the regression task, the final prediction is typically based on the average of the predictions from all the trees [95].

NB:

NB is a classification tool based on Bayes' Theorem and the assumption of feature independence. Various variants of Naive Bayes exist in the literature, each with different application properties. The most widely used versions include Gaussian Naive Bayes (for continuous data), Multinomial Naive Bayes (for discrete data), Bernoulli Naive Bayes (for binary data), and HNB (Hidden Naive Bayes). The core idea revolves around calculating the conditional probability of an event, given prior information. The mathematical expression of Bayes theorem is:

$$P(A|B) = \frac{P(B|A)P(A)}{P(B)}, \tag{3.1}$$

where A and B are events, and $P(B) \neq 0$. Using a dataset example, Bayes' Theorem in classification tasks works as follows:

$$P(y|X) = \frac{P(X|y)P(y)}{P(X)}, \tag{3.2}$$

where y is a class variable and X is the dependent feature vector as presented $X = (x_1, x_2, \ldots, x_n)$. Here, $P(y|X)$ is the probability class of y given the data X, known as posterior probability. $P(X|y)$ is the likelihood of data given class C. $P(y)$ is the prior probability of class y and $P(X)$ is the probability of the data X. In AI applications, Naive Bayes is commonly used for classification tasks. The final expression becomes: $P(y|X) \propto P(y) \cdot P(x_1|y) \cdot P(x_2|y) \ldots, P(x_n|y)$, and the class y that maximizes this expression is the predicted class [96, 97].

LR:

LR is a widely used classification technique, particularly effective with medical datasets [98]. It classifies data into discrete categories by learning relationships from labelled data. LR captures a linear relationship from the dataset and introduces nonlinearity through an activation function to establish a hyperplane that separates data points into two distinct classes. The logistic function is the most used activation function in LR for binary classification tasks. The method focuses on finding the optimal hyperplane or decision boundary that divides the observed data into two categories. The sigmoid function, a mathematical function, takes input from a broad range of values and outputs results between 0 and 1. This function, often used in neural networks as an activation function, helps in processing information. In logistic regression, the sigmoid function transforms the input data into probabilities ranging from 0 to 1, making it ideal for datasets with discrete target variables.

Assume we have exclusively binary or continuous explanatory variables $X = (X_1, X_2, X_{3,\ldots\ldots\ldots} X_m)^t$ where X^t is the transpose of X and Y is a binary response variable. The values of Y divide the possible values of X into two distinct subsets, X_0 and X_1, which are separated by an affine hyperplane $\mathscr{h} \subset \mathbb{R}^m$. The cartesian equation of h is defined by $m + 1$ real parameters $\mathscr{w} = (\mathscr{w}_0, \ldots, \mathscr{w}_m)^t$, such that for any all $x = (x_1, x_2, x_3, \ldots, x_m)^t \in \mathbb{R}^m$, the conditions for being on the hyperplane is:

$$x \in \mathscr{h} \Leftrightarrow \mathscr{w}_0, \mathscr{w}_1 x_1, \ldots, +\mathscr{w}_m x_m = 0. \tag{3.3}$$

In practice, the two subsets $\mathcal{X}_1$ and $\mathcal{X}_0$ are not always perfectly separated by an affine hyperplane but rather by a more complex hypersurface. As a result, this model may produce both false positive and false negative predictions. By $X(\Omega)$ using an affine hyperplane, we can define the following classification regions:

$\chi_1 = \{x \in \mathbb{R}^m | \mathscr{w}_0, \mathscr{w}_1 x_1, \ldots, +\mathscr{w}_m x_m| > 0\}$, which corresponds to the class where $Y = 1$. $\chi_0 = \{x \in \mathbb{R}^m | \mathscr{w}_0, \mathscr{w}_1 x_1, \ldots, +\mathscr{w}_m x_m| \leq 0\}$, which corresponds to the class where $Y = 0$.

For a given observation $X \in X(\Omega)$,,, the random variable $[Y|X = x]$ follows Bernoulli distribution with parameters $S_W(X)$, i.e., $[Y|X = x] \rightarrow \mathcal{B}(S_w(x))$. The probability that $Y = 1$ given $X = x$ is:

$\mathbb{P}(Y = 1|X = x) = S_w(x)$, where $\mathbb{P}(A)$ denotes the probability of event A, and $S_W(\cdot)$ is a score function that maps $\mathbb{R}^m$ to [0,1].

Given a threshold $\theta \in [0, 1]$, the classification rule is as follows:

- $x \in \mathcal{X}_1$ if $S_w(x) \geq \theta$, and
- $x \in \mathcal{X}_1$ if $S_w(x) < \theta$.

A typical threshold value is $\theta = 0.5$, but stricter classification can be applied by choosing $\theta > 0.5$. For the logistic model, the score function $S_w(x)$ is defined as: $S_w(x) = \sigma(w_0, w_1 x_1, \ldots, +w_m x_m)$, where $\sigma(x) = \frac{1}{1+\exp(-x)}$ is a sigmoid function [99].

k-NN:

It is a straightforward classification approach, which is worked based on the class of their nearest neighbours. It is often useful to take more than one neighbour into account, so the technique is more commonly referred to as k-NN Classification, where k-nearest neighbours is used in determining the class. Let's assume that the training dataset D is made up of $(x_i)_{i\in[1,n]}$ training samples (where $n = |D|$). The examples are described by a set of features F and any numeric features have been normalized to the change [0,1]. Each training example is labelled with a class label $y_j \in Y$. The prime goal is to classify an unknown example q. For each $x_i \in D$. Now calculation of the distance between two points is estimated by Euclidean distance. Then there is a variety of ways in which the k-nearest neighbours can be used to determine the class of q. The most straightforward approach is to assign the majority class among the nearest neighbours to the query. A general technique to achieve this is distance-weighted voting, where the neighbours get to vote on the class of the query case with votes weighted by the inverse of their distance to the query.

$$\text{Vote } (y_i) = \sum_{c=1}^{k} \frac{1}{(q, x_c)^p} 1\left(y_j, y_c\right). \tag{3.4}$$

Thus, the vote assigned to a class y_j by neighbour x_c is 1 divided by the distance to that neighbour, i.e., $1(y_j, y_c)$ returns 1 if the class labels match and 0 otherwise. Here, the value of P is varied. Another way to voting is based on Shepard's work and uses an exponential function rather than inverse distance,

$$\text{Vote}(y_i) = \sum_{c=1}^{k} e^{d(q,x_c)} 1\left(y_j, y_c\right). \tag{3.5}$$

Voting is used for classification, whereas K-NN also worked well for regression [100].

MLP:

An MLP is a type of FNN where information flows in a single direction through the network. In this architecture, the neurons are arranged in multiple parallel layers. The first layer is known as the input layer, while the last layer is referred to as the output layer; the layers in between are called hidden layers. When an FNN contains only one hidden layer, it is specifically termed an MLP [101]. Based on the weights, inputs, and biases, the outputs of the MLP are evaluated through the following steps: First, the weighted sum is calculated as follows:

$$a_i = \sum_{j=1}^{n} (Y_{ji}, Z_j) - Y_{a+1}, \quad \text{and} \quad i = 1, 2, \ldots, c, \tag{3.6}$$

where n denotes the number of input nodes, Y_{ji} represents the association weight's accuracy from the jth node the reby corresponding to the input layer of the ith node corresponding to the hidden layer, Z_j represents the input j, c denotes the count of hidden nodes and Y_{a+1} is the threshold value of the hidden node i. The individual hidden node's output is calculated by the following equation:

$$P_i = sig\ M(a_i) = {}^1/_{(1 + \exp(-a_i))}, \quad i = 1, 2, \ldots, c. \tag{3.7}$$

The overall outputs are categorized based on the hidden node's evaluated outputs.

$$r_s = \sum_{i=1}^{s} (Y_{is}, P_i) - D'_s, \quad s = 1, 2, \ldots, n. \tag{3.8}$$

Thus, the output of MLP has been found via the bias weights.

$$H_s = sig\ M(r_s) = {}^1/_{(1 + \exp(-r_s))}, \quad k = 1,\ 2 \ldots,\ n. \tag{3.9}$$

ANNs:

An ANN is a computational model inspired by biological systems, consisting of numerous interconnected units known as artificial neurons. These units, also called processing elements (PEs), are connected by coefficients referred to as weights, which shape the network's structure. Each PE processes information through weighted inputs, a transfer function, and a single output, effectively operating as an equation that balances inputs and outputs. ANNs are often termed connectionist models because the connection weights serve as the system's memory. While a single neuron can manage basic information-processing tasks, the true strength of neural computations emerges from the interconnectedness of multiple neurons within a network. The debate regarding whether artificial neural networks possess intelligence comparable to that of humans continues. ANNs typically consist of only a few hundred to a few thousand PEs, whereas the human brain contains approximately 100 billion neurons. As a result, artificial networks that match the brain's complexity are still far from achieving its creative capabilities. The human brain is considerably more complex, and many of its cognitive functions remain not fully understood. Nonetheless, ANNs can process large volumes of data and make surprisingly accurate predictions, though this ability does not equate to intelligence in the traditional human sense; thus, the term "computer intelligence" may be more appropriate for these systems. In the literature, various types of ANNs are documented according to their application areas. When utilizing neural networks for data analysis, it is essential to distinguish between ANN models (the architecture of the network) and ANN algorithms (the computations that produce the network's outputs). Once the network has been designed for a specific application, it is ready for training, which can be approached in two main ways: supervised and unsupervised learning. The most used ANN is a fully connected, supervised network that employs the backpropagation learning rule, excelling in prediction and classification tasks. Furthermore, the Kohonen network, or Self-Organizing Map, utilizes an unsupervised learning algorithm and is particularly effective at uncovering relationships within complex datasets [102].

Ensemble Tools:

The primary objective of ensemble methods is to reduce the misclassification rate of weak classifiers by aggregating multiple classifiers. The basic idea is to obtain predictions from various classifiers on the original data and combine these predictions to create a strong classifier. As a result, overfitting issues are reduced, and performance on unseen data is improved. By this approach, ensemble methods can enhance the robustness and generalization of machine learning models. Here, we discuss the widely used ensemble methods in healthcare for prediction and classification.

ADA:

ADA is an ensemble learning technique that operates iteratively, leveraging the errors of weak classifiers that perform just slightly better than random guessing and enhancing their effectiveness to transform them into strong classifiers. The core of AdaBoost lies in its ability to combine multiple weak classifiers, increasing the weights of those that demonstrate superior performance. While AdaBoost was not specifically designed for imbalanced datasets, its tendency to assign greater weights to underrepresented classes makes it a promising approach for addressing classification issues in such contexts. This focus helps the algorithm accurately categorize these less-represented samples. However, extremely skewed class distributions can still pose challenges for this method.

The fundamental works as follows. Given a training set $(X, Y) = \{(x_1, y_1) \ldots, (x_N, y_N)|x_i \in R^d, y_i \in \{-1, +1\}, i = 1, \ldots, N$, where x_i is the feature vector of i-th example and y_i is its class label. The weights for all examples are initialized uniformly by $w_i \leftarrow w_i \cdot \exp(-y_i f_m(x_i))/z$ with the normalized factor Z which is defined by $Z = \sum_{i=1}^{N} w_i$. At each boosting iteration, a new weak classifier is added, and the process is repeated until a certain stopping condition is met (e.g., a predefined number of M weak classifiers are trained). Finally, a strong classifier $F(x)$ is computed as a linear combination of all weak classifiers.

$$F(x) = \sum_{m=1}^{M} f_m(x). \tag{3.10}$$

In object detection, the sign of $F(x)$ decides the prediction object label, while its absolute value is a confidence measure for this prediction. The higher the absolute value is, the more confident is the result [103].

GBT:

The GBT algorithm is a popular ensemble method, like RF, with a key difference: GBT builds decision trees sequentially. Each new tree in the ensemble corrects errors made by previous trees by focusing on their residuals. This sequential process allows GBT to learn intricate relationships within the data, though it also increases the risk of overfitting if not carefully regularized. Common regularization techniques include adjusting the learning rate, limiting tree depth, setting a minimum number of samples per leaf, and applying subsampling. By combining these techniques, a well-regularized GBT model can generalize effectively to new data, often achieving higher predictive accuracy, though it may be more sensitive to noisy data. The mathematical foundation of GBT relies on more than just regularization techniques. Several key concepts are involved, including loss function minimization, additive model structure, gradient descent for error minimization, tree fitting on residuals, and prediction updates. In most cases, loss function minimization uses Mean Squared Error for regression or logarithmic loss for classification, depending on the problem type. Additionally, GBT employs gradient descent to sequentially reduce errors by building an additive model of decision trees. Each tree targets the residuals of the previous model, while regularization controls model complexity to ensure effective generalization to unseen data. This approach enables GBT to model complex relationships in data effectively [104].

XGB:

The popular machine learning algorithm XGB is based on gradient-boosted decision trees and is known for its ability to enhance overall model performance while reducing overfitting during training. XGB achieves this with the help of L1 and L2 regularization [105], which improve model generalization and mitigate overfitting. The algorithm uses the second partial derivative of the loss function, providing more detailed information about the gradient's direction for optimization. A key factor in XGB's success is its objective function, which comprises a loss function and a regularization term. The loss function measures the difference between each predicted value and its actual value, while the regularization term controls model complexity to prevent overfitting. Mathematically, the model is defined as: $\hat{Y}_i = \sum_{k=1}^{k} f_k(x_i)$, here final prediction is $\hat{Y}_i$ for an input x_i as the sum of predictions from the multiple DT, and f_k is a DT and K is the total number of trees. Additionally, XGB is often faster than traditional gradient boosting because it can parallelize tree construction, further enhancing efficiency [105].

CBT:

CBT is a powerful and efficient gradient boosting algorithm that excels in handling categorical data and reduces the risk of overfitting, often requiring less tuning compared to other gradient boosting methods. It uses symmetric trees, where each level of the tree has the same split across branches, which speeds up both training and inference. The mathematical foundation of CBT is based on the gradient boosting framework, where the model prediction is defined as: $\hat{y}_i^{(t)} = \hat{y}_j^{(t-1)} + \eta f_t(x_i)$. After t iterations, the model prediction for an instance x_i is iteratively updated by adding a decision tree that reduces the prediction error. The primary objective is to minimize the loss function, with regularization techniques such as L2 regularization and controlling tree complexity (e.g., tree depth and number of leaves) to prevent overfitting. Additionally, hyperparameter tuning and early stopping are other tools used to regulate the model's performance [106].

LGBM:

LGBM is a high-performance, scalable gradient boosting algorithm tailored for large-scale machine learning tasks. By utilizing a histogram-based approach to discretize continuous features, it significantly accelerates training and reduces memory usage. Unlike traditional level-wise growth methods, LGBM employs a leaf-wise tree growth strategy, selecting the leaf that minimizes the loss function. This approach often results in deeper trees and higher accuracy. A key advantage of LGBM is its native support for categorical features, which eliminates the need for complex preprocessing like one-hot encoding. The algorithm is also optimized for efficiency, with support for parallel processing and GPU acceleration, making it an excellent choice for large datasets. This algorithm incorporates regularization techniques, including L1 and L2 regularization, and provides parameters to control tree depth and leaf complexity, which help mitigate overfitting. Its combination of speed, flexibility, and accuracy has made it a popular choice for classification and regression tasks alike. Built on the principles of gradient boosting, LGBM aims to minimize the loss function through its histogram-based discretization and leaf-wise tree-building approach, delivering fast and scalable performance even on very large datasets [107].

3.6 Challenges and Considerations

The integration of AI into healthcare presents significant opportunities to transform diagnostics, treatment personalization, and operational efficiency, but its successful implementation faces multiple complex challenges. One major concern involves data security and privacy, as healthcare AI systems must handle sensitive patient information while mitigating risks of re-identification and cybersecurity threats. Additionally, algorithmic bias remains a critical issue, with many models producing skewed or inequitable outcomes due to unrepresentative training data, highlighting the need for robust bias detection and mitigation strategies. The inherent opacity of many AI systems also creates transparency barriers, limiting clinician trust and necessitating the development of Explainable AI frameworks. Furthermore, unclear regulatory guidelines and liability structures surrounding AI-assisted diagnostics complicate governance and slow adoption. Beyond other critical obstacles, technical integration presents significant challenges, particularly due to incompatibility with legacy

EHR systems, which hinders seamless implementation. Physician resistance further complicates adoption, stemming from concerns about job displacement, excessive reliance on automated systems, and perceived loss of clinical autonomy. Additional limitations emerge from AI systems' inability to generalize across diverse healthcare environments and their challenges with continuous learning, including risks of catastrophic forgetting and model instability. These technical barriers are compounded by economic disparities and the digital divide, which create unequal access to AI technologies and risk widening existing healthcare inequities. Concurrent ethical concerns regarding informed consent processes and the potential erosion of clinical judgment require careful consideration.

Additionally, real-world examples highlight both the potential and challenges of AI in healthcare. IBM Watson Health failed to gain widespread adoption due to discrepancies between its training data and real-world clinical workflows in oncology, ultimately leading to its shutdown [108]. Similarly, an AI-based sepsis prediction tool exhibited racial bias by underestimating risk for black patients, a flaw stemming from biased training data [109]. In contrast, Google's DeepMind system demonstrated expert-level accuracy in detecting diabetic retinopathy but faced challenges in integrating with diverse healthcare infrastructures [110]. The Epic Deterioration Index, used extensively during the COVID-19 pandemic, was criticized for potential racial bias in patient risk assessments [111].

Moreover, to successfully overcome these challenges, a dual-focused strategy is essential, one that harmonizes technological advancement with rigorous ethical standards. This balanced approach must ensure AI implementations augment rather than disrupt clinical workflows while safeguarding patient welfare and maintaining public confidence. Achieving this goal requires concerted collaboration across disciplines, uniting computer scientists, healthcare providers, bioethicists, and government regulators to create holistic governance structures. Together, these stakeholders must develop adaptable frameworks that promote both innovation and responsibility, enabling the safe, clinically validated, and equitable deployment of AI technologies throughout healthcare systems. Such comprehensive solutions will need to address technical limitations while upholding fundamental medical ethics, ultimately fostering AI applications that enhance rather than replace human clinical judgment and equitable care delivery.

3.7 Conclusion

Integrating AI into healthcare holds immense potential to revolutionize diagnostics, personalize treatments, and streamline operations. However, realizing these benefits requires addressing critical challenges, including data privacy concerns, algorithmic biases, regulatory ambiguity, and technical integration hurdles. Ensuring that AI systems are safe, fair, and effective demands a coordinated effort among technologists, clinicians, ethicists, and policymakers. Such collaboration is key to developing strong governance models, enhancing model transparency, reducing bias, and promoting equitable access across various healthcare environments. By committing to ethical AI design, ongoing validation, and inclusive stakeholder involvement, the healthcare sector can unlock AI's transformative power while maintaining patient trust and ensuring fair, widespread impact.

References

1. Hamet, P., & Tremblay, J. (2017). Artificial intelligence in medicine. *Metabolism, 69*, S36–S40.
2. Kaul, V., Enslin, S., & Gross, S. A. (2020). History of artificial intelligence in medicine. *Gastrointestinal Endoscopy, 92*(4), 807–812.
3. Briganti, G., & Le Moine, O. (2020). Artificial intelligence in medicine: Today and tomorrow. *Frontiers in Medicine, 7*, 27.
4. Knight, B. A., Potretzke, A. M., Larson, J. A., & Bhayani, S. B. (2015). Comparing expert reported outcomes to national surgical quality improvement program risk calculator-predicted outcomes: Do reporting standards differ? *Journal of Endourology, 29*(9), 1091–1099.
5. Destephe, M., Brandao, M., Kishi, T., Zecca, M., Hashimoto, K., & Takanishi, A. (2015). Walking in the uncanny valley: Importance of the attractiveness on the acceptance of a robot as a working partner. *Frontiers in Psychology, 6*, 204.
6. Haleem, A., Javaid, M., & Khan, I. H. (2019). Current status and applications of Artificial Intelligence (AI) in medical field: An overview. *Current Medicine Research and Practice, 9*(6), 231–237.
7. Ellahham, S., Ellahham, N., & Simsekler, M. C. E. (2020). Application of artificial intelligence in the health care safety context: Opportunities and challenges. *American Journal of Medical Quality, 35*(4), 341–348.
8. Capaccione, K. M., & Salvatore, M. M. (2023). Radiographic grading system for usual interstitial pneumonia correlates with mortality and may serve as a surrogate endpoint in clinical trials. *Clinical Imaging, 102*, 37–41.
9. Rana, M., & Bhushan, M. (2023). Machine learning and deep learning approach for medical image analysis: Diagnosis to detection. *Multimedia Tools and Applications, 82*(17), 26731–26769.
10. Sharma, P., Malik, S., Sehgal, S., & Pruthi, J. (2013). Computer aided diagnosis based on medical image processing and artificial intelligence methods. *International Journal of Information and Computation Technology, 3*(9), 887–892.
11. Han, X., & Xu, W. (2021). Research on medical image diagnosis method based on artificial intelligence. *International Journal of Frontiers in Medicine, 3*(2).
12. Muthuraju, V., Manur, D., Farook, M. F., KS, C. G., & Desai, S. M. (2021, August). Doctor patient assistance system using artificial intelligence. In *2021 second international conference on electronics and sustainable communication systems (ICESC)* (pp. 534–538). IEEE.
13. Kocaballi, A. B., Ijaz, K., Laranjo, L., Quiroz, J. C., Rezazadegan, D., Tong, H. L., et al. (2020). Envisioning an artificial intelligence documentation assistant for future primary care consultations: A co-design study with general practitioners. *Journal of the American Medical Informatics Association, 27*(11), 1695–1704.
14. Eriksson, P., Hammar, T., Lagrosen, S., & Nilsson, E. (2022). Digital consultation in primary healthcare: The effects on access, efficiency and patient safety based on provider experience; a qualitative study. *Scandinavian Journal of Primary Health Care, 40*(4), 498–506.
15. Mehraeen, E., SeyedAlinaghi, S., Heydari, M., Karimi, A., Mahdavi, A., Mashoufi, M., Sarmad, A., Mirghaderi, P., Shamsabadi, A., Qaderi, K., Mirzapour, P., & Noori, T. (2023). Telemedicine technologies and applications in the era of COVID-19 pandemic: A systematic review. *Health informatics journal, 29*(2), 14604582231167431.

16. Kumar, Y., Koul, A., Singla, R., & Ijaz, M. F. (2023). Artificial intelligence in disease diagnosis: A systematic literature review, synthesizing framework and future research agenda. *Journal of Ambient Intelligence and Humanized Computing, 14*(7), 8459–8486.
17. Ghaffar Nia, N., Kaplanoglu, E., & Nasab, A. (2023). Evaluation of artificial intelligence techniques in disease diagnosis and prediction. *Discover Artificial Intelligence, 3*(1), 5.
18. Mathis-Ullrich, F., & Scheikl, P. M. (2021). Robots in the operating room—(co) operation during surgery. *Der Gastroenterologe, 16*, 25–34.
19. Probst, P. (2023). A review of the role of robotics in surgery: To DaVinci and beyond! *Missouri Medicine, 120*(5), 389–396.
20. Qiu, Y., Ashok, A., Nguyen, C. C., Yamauchi, Y., Do, T. N., & Phan, H. P. (2024). Integrated sensors for soft medical robotics. *Small*, 2308805.
21. Lefetz, O., Baste, J. M., Hamel, J. F., Mordojovich, G., Lefevre-Scelles, A., & Coq, J. M. (2024). Robotic surgery and work-related stress: A systematic review. *Applied Ergonomics, 117*, Article 104188.
22. Walia, N., Zahedi, F. M., & Jain, H. (2017). Potential of virtual worlds for nursing care: lessons and outcomes. *OJIN: The Online Journal of Issues in Nursing, 23*(1).
23. Huun, K. (2018). Virtual simulations in online nursing education: Align with quality matters. *Clinical Simulation in Nursing, 22*, 26–31.
24. Ngayua, E. N., He, J., & Agyei-Boahene, K. (2021). Applying advanced technologies to improve clinical trials: A systematic mapping study. *Scientometrics, 126*(2), 1217–1238.
25. Askin, S., Burkhalter, D., Calado, G., & El Dakrouni, S. (2023). Artificial intelligence applied to clinical trials: Opportunities and challenges. *Health and Technology, 13*(2), 203–213. https://doi.org/10.1007/s12553-023-00738-2
26. Li, J., Ma, Q., Chan, A. H., & Man, S. (2019). Health monitoring through wearable technologies for older adults: Smart wearables acceptance model. *Applied Ergonomics, 75*, 162–169.
27. Dunn, J., Runge, R., & Snyder, M. (2018). Wearables and the medical revolution. *Personalized Medicine, 15*(5), 429–448.
28. Majumder, S., Mondal, T., & Deen, M. J. (2017). Wearable sensors for remote health monitoring. *Sensors, 17*(1), 130.
29. Knevel, R., & Liao, K. P. (2023). From real-world electronic health record data to real-world results using artificial intelligence. *Annals of the Rheumatic Diseases, 82*(3), 306–311.
30. Goetz, L. H., & Schork, N. J. (2018). Personalized medicine: Motivation, challenges, and progress. *Fertility and Sterility, 109*(6), 952–963.
31. Menachemi, N., & Collum, T. H. (2011). Benefits and drawbacks of electronic health record systems. *Risk management and healthcare policy* (pp. 47–55).
32. Zainal, N. H., Bossarte, R. M., Gildea, S. M., Hwang, I., Kennedy, C. J., Liu, H., Luedtke, A., Marx, B. P., Petukhova, M. V., Post, E. P., Ross, E. L., & Kessler, R. C. (2024). Developing an individualized treatment rule for Veterans with major depressive disorder using electronic health records. *Molecular psychiatry* (pp. 1–11).
33. Wang, Y. F., Chen, Y. C., & Chien, S. Y. (2023). Citizens' intention to follow recommendations from a government-supported AI-enabled system. *Public Policy and Administration*, 09520767231176126.
34. Monarcha-Matlak, A. (2021). Automated decision-making in public administration. *Procedia Computer Science, 192*, 2077–2084.
35. Alyass, A., Turcotte, M., & Meyre, D. (2015). From big data analysis to personalized medicine for all: Challenges and opportunities. *BMC Medical Genomics, 8*, 1–12.
36. Mirbabaie, M., Stieglitz, S., & Frick, N. R. (2021). Artificial intelligence in disease diagnostics: A critical review and classification on the current state of research guiding future direction. *Health and Technology, 11*(4), 693–731.
37. Behara, K., Bhero, E., Agee, J. T., & Gonela, V. (2022). Artificial intelligence in medical diagnostics: A review from a South African context. *Scientific African, 17*, Article e01360.
38. Tripathi, M. K., Nath, A., Singh, T. P., Ethayathulla, A. S., & Kaur, P. (2021). Evolving scenario of big data and artificial intelligence (AI) in drug discovery. *Molecular Diversity, 25*, 1439–1460.

39. Mak, K. K., Wong, Y. H., & Pichika, M. R. (2023). Artificial intelligence in drug discovery and development. *Drug Discovery and Evaluation: Safety and Pharmacokinetic Assays*, 1–38.
40. Blanco-Gonzalez, A., Cabezon, A., Seco-Gonzalez, A., Conde-Torres, D., Antelo-Riveiro, P., Pineiro, A., & Garcia-Fandino, R. (2023). The role of AI in drug discovery: Challenges, opportunities, and strategies. *Pharmaceuticals, 16*(6), 891.
41. Jiménez-Luna, J., Grisoni, F., Weskamp, N., & Schneider, G. (2021). Artificial intelligence in drug discovery: Recent advances and future perspectives. *Expert Opinion on Drug Discovery, 16*(9), 949–959.
42. Reddy, S., Rogers, W., Makinen, V. P., Coiera, E., Brown, P., Wenzel, M., Weicken, E., Ansari, S., Mathur, P., Casey, A., & Kelly, B. (2021). Evaluation framework to guide implementation of AI systems into healthcare settings. *BMJ Health & Care Informatics, 28*(1).
43. oo, I., Alafaireet, P., Marinov, M., Pena-Hernandez, K., Gopidi, R., Chang, J. F., & Hua, L. (2012). Data mining in healthcare and biomedicine: a survey of the literature. *Journal of Medical Systems, 36*, 2431–2448.
44. Kostkova, P., Brewer, H., De Lusignan, S., Fottrell, E., Goldacre, B., Hart, G., Koczan, P., Knight, P., Marsolier, C., McKendry, R. A., Ross, E., & Tooke, J. (2016). Who owns the data? Open data for healthcare. *Frontiers in Public Health, 4*, 7.
45. Krzywicki, T., Brona, P., Zbrzezny, A. M., & Grzybowski, A. E. (2023). A global review of publicly available datasets containing fundus images: Characteristics, barriers to access, usability, and generalizability. *Journal of Clinical Medicine, 12*(10), 3587.
46. Kim, H. (2022). Artificial intelligence ecosystem, techniques, and use cases. *Artificial Intelligence for 6G* (pp. 15–33). Springer International Publishing.
47. Khan, M. R. (2024). Advances in architectures for deep learning: A thorough examination of present trends. *Journal of Artificial Intelligence General Science (JAIGS), 1*(1), 24–30. ISSN: 3006-4023.
48. Vandersluis, R., & Savulescu, J. (2024). The selective deployment of AI in healthcare: An ethical algorithm for algorithms. *Bioethics.*
49. Pickhardt, P. J., Correale, L., & Hassan, C. (2023). AI-based opportunistic CT screening of incidental cardiovascular disease, osteoporosis, and sarcopenia: Cost-effectiveness analysis. *Abdominal Radiology, 48*(3), 1181–1198.
50. Milne-Ives, M., de Cock, C., Lim, E., Shehadeh, M. H., de Pennington, N., Mole, G., Normando, E., & Meinert, E. (2020). The effectiveness of artificial intelligence conversational agents in health care: systematic review. *Journal of Medical Internet Research, 22*(10), e20346.
51. Güell, E. (2024). Criteria for implementing artificial intelligence systems in reproductive medicine. *Clinical and Experimental Reproductive Medicine, 51*(1), 1.
52. Altmann, A., Toloşi, L., Sander, O., & Lengauer, T. (2010). Permutation importance: A corrected feature importance measure. *Bioinformatics, 26*(10), 1340–1347.
53. Rodríguez-Pérez, R., & Bajorath, J. (2021). Feature importance correlation from machine learning indicates functional relationships between proteins and similar compound binding characteristics. *Scientific Reports, 11*(1), 14245.
54. GhoshRoy, D., Alvi, P. A., & Santosh, K. C. (2023, March). Unboxing industry-standard AI models for male fertility prediction with SHAP. In *Healthcare* (Vol. 11, No. 7, p. 929). MDPI.
55. Parr, T., Hamrick, J., & Wilson, J. D. (2024). Nonparametric feature impact and importance. *Information Sciences, 653*, Article 119563.
56. Cunningham, P., & Delany, S. J. (2021). Underestimation bias and underfitting in machine learning. In *Trustworthy AI-Integrating Learning, Optimization and Reasoning: First International Workshop, TAILOR 2020, Virtual Event, September 4–5, 2020, Revised Selected Papers 1* (pp. 20–31). Springer International Publishing.
57. Mehrotra, R., Ansari, M. A., Agrawal, R., & Anand, R. S. (2020). A transfer learning approach for AI-based classification of brain tumors. *Machine Learning with Applications, 2*, Article 100003.
58. Buchlak, Q. D., Esmaili, N., Leveque, J. C., Bennett, C., Farrokhi, F., & Piccardi, M. (2021). Machine learning applications to neuroimaging for glioma detection and classification: An

artificial intelligence augmented systematic review. *Journal of Clinical Neuroscience, 89*, 177–198.
59. Shipe, M. E., Deppen, S. A., Farjah, F., & Grogan, E. L. (2019). Developing prediction models for clinical use using logistic regression: An overview. *Journal of Thoracic Disease, 11*(Suppl 4), S574.
60. Curchoe, C. L., Farias, A. F. S., Mendizabal-Ruiz, G., & Chavez-Badiola, A. (2020). Evaluating predictive models in reproductive medicine. *Fertility and Sterility, 114*(5), 921–926.
61. Wang, R., Pan, W., Jin, L., Li, Y., Geng, Y., Gao, C., Chen, G., Wang, H., Ma, D., & Liao, S. (2019). Artificial intelligence in reproductive medicine. *Reproduction, 158*(4), R139–R154.
62. Kelly, C. J., Karthikesalingam, A., Suleyman, M., Corrado, G., & King, D. (2019). Key challenges for delivering clinical impact with artificial intelligence. *BMC Medicine, 17*, 1–9.
63. Zhao, Z. A., & Liu, H. (2012). *Spectral feature selection for data mining*. Taylor & Francis.
64. Russell, S. J., & Norvig, P. (2016). *Artificial intelligence: A modern approach*. Pearson.
65. Guyon, I., Gunn, S., Nikravesh, M., & Zadeh, L. A. (Eds.). (2008). *Feature extraction: Foundations and applications* (Vol. 207). Springer.
66. Saeys, Y., Abeel, T., & Van de Peer, Y. (2008). Robust feature selection using ensemble feature selection techniques. In *Machine learning and knowledge discovery in databases: European conference, ECML PKDD 2008, Antwerp, Belgium, September 15–19, 2008, proceedings, Part II 19* (pp. 313–325). Springer.
67. Bolón-Canedo, V., Sánchez-Maroño, N., & Alonso-Betanzos, A. (2010, July). On the effectiveness of discretization on gene selection of microarray data. In *The 2010 international joint conference on neural networks (IJCNN)* (pp. 1–8). IEEE.
68. Kohavi, R., & John, G. H. (1997). Wrappers for feature subset selection. *Artificial Intelligence, 97*(1–2), 273–324.
69. Pudjihartono, N., Fadason, T., Kempa-Liehr, A. W., & O'Sullivan, J. M. (2022). A review of feature selection methods for machine learning-based disease risk prediction. *Frontiers in Bioinformatics, 2*, Article 927312.
70. Hall, M. A. (1999). *Correlation-based feature selection for machine learning* (Doctoral dissertation, The University of Waikato).
71. Yoshida, M., & Koike, A. (2011). SNPInterForest: A new method for detecting epistatic interactions. *BMC Bioinformatics, 12*, 1–10.
72. Dash, M., & Liu, H. (2003). Consistency-based search in feature selection. *Artificial Intelligence, 151*(1–2), 155–176.
73. Zhao, Z., & Liu, H. (2009). Searching for interacting features in subset selection. *Intelligent Data Analysis, 13*(2), 207–228.
74. Hall, M. A., & Smith, L. A. (1998). Practical feature subset selection for machine learning.
75. Kira, K., & Rendell, L. A. (1992, July). The feature selection problem: Traditional methods and a new algorithm. In *Proceedings of the tenth national conference on Artificial intelligence* (pp. 129–134).
76. Guyon, I., Weston, J., Barnhill, S., & Vapnik, V. (2002). Gene selection for cancer classification using support vector machines. *Machine Learning, 46*, 389–422.
77. Bolón-Canedo, V., Sánchez-Maroño, N., & Alonso-Betanzos, A. (2013). A review of feature selection methods on synthetic data. *Knowledge and Information Systems, 34*, 483–519.
78. Ghosh, M., Guha, R., Sarkar, R., & Abraham, A. (2020). A wrapper-filter feature selection technique based on ant colony optimization. *Neural Computing and Applications, 32*, 7839–7857.
79. Kononenko, I. (1994, April). Estimating attributes: Analysis and extensions of RELIEF. In *European conference on machine learning* (pp. 171–182). Springer.
80. Jain, R., & Xu, W. (2023). Artificial Intelligence based wrapper for high dimensional feature selection. *BMC Bioinformatics, 24*(1), 392.
81. Herold, C., Steffens, M., Brockschmidt, F. F., Baur, M. P., & Becker, T. (2009). INTERSNP: Genome-wide interaction analysis guided by a priori information. *Bioinformatics, 25*(24), 3275–3281.

82. Pes, B. (2020). Ensemble feature selection for high-dimensional data: A stability analysis across multiple domains. *Neural Computing and Applications, 32*(10), 5951–5973.
83. Jothi, G. (2016). Hybrid tolerance rough set-firefly based supervised feature selection for MRI brain tumor image classification. *Applied Soft Computing, 46*, 639–651.
84. Hernández-Pereira, E., Bolón-Canedo, V., Sánchez-Maroño, N., Álvarez-Estévez, D., Moret-Bonillo, V., & Alonso-Betanzos, A. (2016). A comparison of performance of K-complex classification methods using feature selection. *Information Sciences, 328*, 1–14.
85. Radovic, M., Ghalwash, M., Filipovic, N., & Obradovic, Z. (2017). Minimum redundancy maximum relevance feature selection approach for temporal gene expression data. *BMC Bioinformatics, 18*, 1–14.
86. Balendran, A., Beji, C., Bouvier, F., Khalifa, O., Evgeniou, T., Ravaud, P., & Porcher, R. (2025). A scoping review of robustness concepts for machine learning in healthcare. *npj Digital Medicine, 8*(1), 38.
87. He, H., & Garcia, E. A. (2009). Learning from imbalanced data. *IEEE Transactions on Knowledge and Data Engineering, 21*(9), 1263–1284.
88. Salmi, M., Atif, D., Oliva, D., Abraham, A., & Ventura, S. (2024). Handling imbalanced medical datasets: Review of a decade of research. *Artificial Intelligence Review, 57*(10), 273.
89. Stitson, M. O., Weston, J. A. E., Gammerman, A., Vovk, V., & Vapnik, V. (1996). Theory of support vector machines. *University of London, 117*(827), 188–191.
90. Huang, M. W., Chen, C. W., Lin, W. C., Ke, S. W., & Tsai, C. F. (2017). SVM and SVM ensembles in breast cancer prediction. *PLoS ONE, 12*(1), Article e0161501.
91. Hassan, M. R., Al-Insaif, S., Hossain, M. I., & Kamruzzaman, J. (2020). A machine learning approach for prediction of pregnancy outcome following IVF treatment. *Neural Computing and Applications, 32*(7), 2283–2297.
92. Tran, T. O., & Le, N. Q. K. (2024). Sa-ttca: An svm-based approach for tumor t-cell antigen classification using features extracted from biological sequencing and natural language processing. *Computers in Biology and Medicine, 174*, Article 108408.
93. Patel, N., & Upadhyay, S. (2012). Study of various decision tree pruning methods with their empirical comparison in WEKA. *International Journal of Computer Applications, 60*(12).
94. Klusowski, J. M., & Tian, P. M. (2024). Large scale prediction with decision trees. *Journal of the American Statistical Association, 119*(545), 525–537.
95. Yadav, A., Singh, A., Dutta, M. K., & Travieso, C. M. (2020). Machine learning-based classification of cardiac diseases from PCG recorded heart sounds. *Neural Computing and Applications, 32*(24), 17843–17856.
96. Al-Taie, R. R. K., Saleh, B. J., Saedi, A. Y. F., & Salman, L. A. (2021). Analysis of WEKA data mining algorithms Bayes net, random forest, MLP and SMO for heart disease prediction system: A case study in Iraq. *International Journal of Electrical and Computer Engineering, 11*(6), 5229.
97. Webb, G. I., Keogh, E., & Miikkulainen, R. (2010). Naïve Bayes. *Encyclopedia of Machine Learning, 15*(1), 713–714.
98. Dreiseitl, S., & Ohno-Machado, L. (2002). Logistic regression and artificial neural network classification models: A methodology review. *Journal of biomedical informatics, 35*(5–6), 352–359.
99. Zaidi, A., & Al Luhayb, A. S. M. (2023). Two statistical approaches to justify the use of the logistic function in binary logistic regression. *Mathematical Problems in Engineering, 2023*(1), 5525675.
100. Guo, G., Wang, H., Bell, D., Bi, Y., & Greer, K. (2003). KNN model-based approach in classification. In *On the move to meaningful internet systems 2003: CoopIS, DOA, and ODBASE: OTM confederated international conferences, CoopIS, DOA, and ODBASE 2003, Catania, Sicily, Italy, November 3-7, 2003. Proceedings* (pp. 986–996). Springer.
101. Deepika, D., & Balaji, N. (2022). Effective heart disease prediction using novel MLP-EBMDA approach. *Biomedical Signal Processing and Control, 72*, Article 103318.
102. Agatonovic-Kustrin, S., & Beresford, R. (2000). Basic concepts of artificial neural network (ANN) modeling and its application in pharmaceutical research. *Journal of Pharmaceutical and Biomedical Analysis, 22*(5), 717–727.

103. Schapire, R. E. (2013). Explaining adaboost. In *Empirical inference: Festschrift in honor of vladimir N. Vapnik* (pp. 37–52). Springer.
104. Chen, J., Huang, H., Cohn, A. G., Zhang, D., & Zhou, M. (2022). Machine learning-based classification of rock discontinuity trace: SMOTE oversampling integrated with GBT ensemble learning. *International Journal of Mining Science and Technology, 32*(2), 309–322.
105. Pathy, A., Meher, S., & Balasubramanian, P. (2020). Predicting algal biochar yield using eXtreme Gradient Boosting (XGB) algorithm of machine learning methods. *Algal Research, 50*, Article 102006.
106. Hancock, J. T., & Khoshgoftaar, T. M. (2020). CatBoost for big data: An interdisciplinary review. *Journal of Big Data, 7*(1), 94.
107. Omotehinwa, T. O., Oyewola, D. O., & Moung, E. G. (2024). Optimizing the light gradient-boosting machine algorithm for an efficient early detection of coronary heart disease. *Informatics and Health, 1*(2), 70–81.
108. Ross, C., & Swetlitz, I. (2018). IBM's Watson supercomputer recommended 'unsafe and incorrect' cancer treatments, internal documents show. *Stat, 25*, 1–10.
109. Wong, A., Otles, E., Donnelly, J. P., Krumm, A., McCullough, J., DeTroyer-Cooley, O., Pestrue, J., Phillips, M., Konye, J., Penoza, C., Ghous, M., & Singh, K. (2021). External validation of a widely implemented proprietary sepsis prediction model in hospitalized patients. *JAMA Internal Medicine, 181*(8), 1065–1070.
110. Gulshan, V., Peng, L., Coram, M., Stumpe, M. C., Wu, D., Narayanaswamy, A., Venugopalan, S., Widner, K., Madams, T., Cuadros, J. and Kim, R., & Webster, D. R. (2016). Development and validation of a deep learning algorithm for detection of diabetic retinopathy in retinal fundus photographs. *jama, 316*(22), 2402–2410.
111. Gianfrancesco, M. A., Tamang, S., Yazdany, J., & Schmajuk, G. (2018). Potential biases in machine learning algorithms using electronic health record data. *JAMA Internal Medicine, 178*(11), 1544–1547.

Chapter 4
Leveraging AI Models/Tools for Human Fertility

4.1 Introduction

In reproductive medicine, conventional methods of therapy typically begin with a detailed assessment of both partners, including several laboratory tests. These procedures are often expensive and time-intensive, contributing to emotional strain and psychological distress. To achieve optimal outcomes over the course of treatment, continuous monitoring and customized adjustments are necessary. However, the demanding nature of the process can lead to increased emotional sensitivity, creating a sense of helplessness and loss of personal agency. In some cases, these emotional burdens may trigger mental health conditions such as anxiety and depression, which can further hinder the chances of conception. To address these challenges, recent years have witnessed the development of innovative treatment strategies aimed at meeting broader population needs. Technological advancements have significantly impacted many fields, particularly through the integration of artificial intelligence. AI has played a transformative role by improving diagnostic accuracy, personalizing treatment approaches, and enhancing the ability to predict outcomes in ART [1].

Traditional protocols such as embryo selection, fertility screening, PCOS, and tumour screening have heavily relied on a clinician's judgment and pre-set criteria. Now, with the implementation of AI, comprehensive datasets such as medical history, hormone readings, imaging, and embryology information can be evaluated to identify hidden patterns that may be beyond human recognition [2]. Additionally, AI supports more efficient decision-making tools for clinicians and helps establish optimized workflows in ART procedures. Therefore, the application of AI tools ultimately aims to enhance the success rates of ART and increase the chances of pregnancy by enabling early identification of fertility-related concerns [3]. Moving forward, as AI continues to evolve, it has the potential to shift the paradigm of reproductive health from a hit-or-miss approach to one driven by data, analytics, and personalized treatment strategies. AI applications extend beyond diagnostic capabilities, particularly in obstetrics and gynecology, enabling advanced monitoring of fetal heart rates and the

KC. Santosh and D. G. Roy, *Artificial Intelligence for Human Fertility: Trends, Insights, and Predictions*, Studies in Computational Intelligence 1230,
https://doi.org/10.1007/978-981-95-1248-5_4

prediction and detection of preterm labour and pregnancy complications. Moreover, exciting new developments such as the individualization of hormone treatments, automated assessment of the uterine lining, and other innovations are anticipated to make reproductive medicine more precise and personalized, ultimately improving outcomes and reducing complications [4].

The integration of artificial intelligence into surgical practice has revolutionized modern gynecological procedures by combining cutting-edge technologies such as high-resolution imaging and micro-operated instrumentation. These advancements have facilitated the widespread adoption of minimally invasive surgery, which is increasingly preferred over traditional open methods due to its association with better outcomes during and after surgery, enhanced patient safety, and improved quality of life, all of which are critical elements in optimizing reproductive health. Robotic-assisted surgery, in particular, offers significant advantages in treating fertility-impacting conditions such as uterine fibroids (leiomyomas), adenomyosis, endometriosis, adnexal masses, sterilization reversal, and fertility preservation procedures. Robotic myomectomy, which has been in clinical use for over a decade, continues to demonstrate strong safety and efficacy profiles [5]. As AI technologies advance, their deeper integration into robotic systems is poised to further enhance surgical precision, minimize complication rates, and improve both short-term patient outcomes and long-term fertility potential.

Despite the numerous exciting technical applications of AI in reproductive medicine and healthcare, a significant challenge remains in determining the most effective and ethical ways to implement AI in clinical practice [6]. AI models depend on large datasets for decision-making, and the quality, diversity, and structure of these datasets are crucial. If data collection strategies are not carefully planned, AI models may inherit or amplify existing biases, which can reduce their effectiveness in certain populations and worsen health disparities. Therefore, researchers and AI scientists working with clinical data must actively identify and address these biases. This can be done by pooling data from multiple centers and diverse sources to create more representative datasets or by clearly acknowledging the limitations of the data and models used. A related concern is the size and representativeness of training datasets, particularly in fields that depend on patient-derived data. While some datasets such as the Human Sperm Head Morphology dataset are publicly available, they are often limited in scale. Barriers such as strict privacy regulations (e.g., HIPAA), the complexity of legacy EHR systems, and institutional competition hinder data sharing across medical centers, making it difficult to assemble large and diverse datasets necessary for robust AI training [7]. However, in fields like oncology and radiology, some of these limitations have been partially overcome through the development of large, shared public datasets. Emerging approaches such as federated learning also offer promising solutions by enabling collaborative model training without the need to share raw patient data, thereby potentially overcoming data-sharing constraints while preserving privacy [8].

Currently, AI research in reproductive medicine primarily focuses on image analysis of sperm cells and embryos, as well as on predicting outcomes of ART. However, applications involving early disease prediction, diagnosis, treatment planning, and prognosis evaluation remain relatively underexplored. Further research is necessary to expand the scope and impact of AI in this field. In certain domains, AI technologies, particularly machine learning models, have matched or even surpassed the performance of expert clinicians. Additionally, the rising concerns about the potential for AI to replace human doctors. It is important to emphasize that AI should be viewed as a tool designed to support and enhance clinical decision-making, not replace it. Machine learning excels at handling simple, repetitive tasks, thereby saving clinicians considerable time and effort. Nonetheless, healthcare professionals must critically assess AI-generated predictions, ensuring that the models are appropriately constructed and aligned with real-world clinical scenarios before applying their outputs in practice [9].

AI is already making significant contributions across various medical specialties, and its influence on reproductive medicine is expected to grow substantially. One particularly promising area is the mechanization of IVF laboratory procedures. The integration of advanced technologies, such as non-subjective sperm and embryo selection, automated oocyte denudation, precise oocyte positioning, fertilization processes, embryo culture, and real-time monitoring of embryo development into fully automated systems, holds the potential to greatly enhance both the efficiency and outcomes of ART. As AI continues to evolve, its development will undoubtedly benefit a larger population of couples facing infertility by improving accessibility, accuracy, and success rates in reproductive care [10].

4.2 AI for Human Fertility Assessment

Studying fertility in humans is challenging, especially given the significant decline observed over the past 50 years. Compounding this issue is the lack of early symptoms, leading many to overlook it as a disease, contributing to a staggering global decline in fertility rates. Research indicates a marked decrease in male fertility, potentially resulting in significant population declines, particularly in developed nations. Therefore, it's crucial to question whether clinical factors alone can explain this decline, as suggested by medical professionals, or if other factors also hold significant influence. The existing infertility epidemic is unquestionably shaped by numerous non-clinical factors like environmental conditions, behavioural patterns, and lifestyle choices. Although these factors may not be directly related to medicine, their widespread impact on human fertility cannot be overlooked [11].

Similar considerations apply to females, who face various gynecological and systemic diseases that can affect their fertility. Lifestyle factors and environmental conditions can exacerbate challenges in conceiving for women. Genetic influences may also limit the number of oocytes in the ovary, delaying attempts at childbearing. Additionally, PCOS is a significant contributor to impaired reproductive function in women. Recent evidence highlights the role of diet, lifestyle, and environment in overcoming ovulatory dysfunction associated with PCOS. Therefore, environmental involvement, lifestyle factors, and diet are crucial factors that impact both males and females [12].

An in-depth analysis reveals that advancing age and obesity are pivotal factors contributing to infertility. The biological mechanisms behind decreased fertility with increasing age are well-documented. Advanced maternal age, for instance, is associated with a heightened risk of unsuccessful pregnancies [13]. Similarly, in males, sperm quality tends to diminish with age, prolonging the time to conception and raising the likelihood of miscarriage and fetal loss [14]. Consequently, as age increases, conception rates tend to decline steadily. Furthermore, obesity has become a prevalent issue, even among teenagers, with profound implications for reproductive health. Not only does obesity compromise oocyte quality, but it also accelerates the aging process and introduces a host of health complications. The rise in obesity can be attributed to factors such as excessive consumption of fast food, sedentary lifestyles, high sugar intake, and disrupted sleep patterns. Despite being overlooked by many, these factors exert significant impacts on human health, particularly on the reproductive system.

In AI-driven landscape, evaluating human fertility has become notably more convenient, especially during the early stages. A plethora of factors are linked with successful pregnancy, serving as essential features in AI-powered fertility assessments. These encompass age, environmental influences, endocrine levels, lifestyle habits, ovarian health, sperm quality, and more. Researchers harness these features to craft potent AI models tailored for fertility assessment. A pivotal aspect of assessing male fertility entails scrutinizing sperm images. These images furnish intricate insights into sperm morphology, often a pivotal determinant in spermatogenesis. Moreover, gauging sperm motility, crucial for effective fertilization, can be accomplished through meticulous image analysis [15]. Researchers amass extensive datasets of sperm images to forge resilient fertility models aimed at discerning male fertility status.

Similarly, in the assessment of female fertility, ultrasound 3-D images assume a critical role, especially in follicular monitoring. These images provide invaluable revelations into ovarian functionality and follicular growth, pivotal for female fertility [16]. By harnessing a multitude of data sources and deploying advanced AI methodologies, researchers can construct intelligent models that serve as indispensable AI-assisted systems for fertility assessment. These models empower clinicians and individuals to gain deeper insights into and manage fertility-related concerns, ultimately fostering enhancements in reproductive health outcomes. In the field of AI, DL and ML algorithms are the primary tools employed. ML methods are utilized to cluster patient features and forecast disease outcomes by scrutinizing structured data like medical imaging and genetic profiles. DL distinguishes itself from traditional ML techniques by its capability to learn complex representations, thereby improving pattern recognition directly from raw data [17].

Unlike conventional ML approaches, DL does not heavily rely on human intervention to organize data or design feature extractors; instead, it autonomously learns from the provided data. Furthermore, alongside ML and DL, there's a burgeoning interest in the adoption of NLP. It plays a pivotal role in converting unstructured data

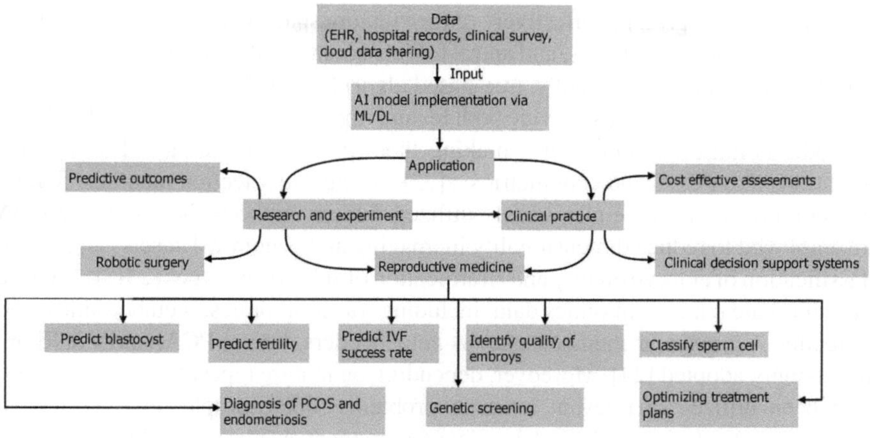

Fig. 4.1 Chart illustrating the application of AI models in medical research and clinical practice. It begins with data sources like EHR, hospital records, and surveys, leading to AI model implementation via machine learning and deep learning. This branches into research and experiment, and clinical practice. Research leads to predictive outcomes, robotic surgery, and reproductive medicine, which further includes predicting blastocyst, fertility, IVF success rate, and diagnosing PCOS and endometriosis. Clinical practice involves cost-effective assessments and clinical decision support systems, focusing on identifying embryo quality, genetic screening, classifying sperm cells, and optimizing treatment plans

into structured formats, allowing machines to comprehend and analyze it using ML techniques [18]. All these techniques are based on mathematical principles and AI-algorithms that enable computers to learn from data and make predictions or decisions without being explicitly programmed for every task. A variety of algorithms are implemented in literature, but based on the problem statement AI researchers opt for a specific solution for their problem. Moreover, Fig. 4.1 illustrates the role of AI in reproductive medicine. Additionally, the following flowchart offers a concise overview of the AI workflow.

4.3 Feature Importance

For reproductive medicine, filter-based feature section methods including mutual information, Pearson correlation, and reliefF are used to identify key clinical and biochemical predictors of outcome such as ovarian response and IVF success. These methods are valued for their computational efficiency and classifier independence [19], though they often overlook complex interactions between features. Furthermore, wrapper methods such as RFE combined classifier like SVM, or LR have been used to improve prediction of embryo viability and live birth outcome by incorporating model performance directly into the feature selection process [20]. Techniques such as LASSO regression effectively reduce feature space while retaining key variables like age, hormone levels, and antral follicle count, producing concise yet meaningful models [21]. Additionally, tree-based algorithms such as random forests and gradient boosting machines provide both feature importance measures and the ability to model nonlinear relationships, making them particularly suitable for complex conditions like PCOS and endometriosis [22]. Alongside selection methods, feature extraction techniques are also widely utilized. Linear methods like PCA and LDA are employed to reduce dimensionality in imaging and genomic datasets, supporting classification of embryo quality and stratification of subfertility types [23]. To capture more intricate patterns in omics data, including transcriptomics, metabolomics, and proteomics—nonlinear methods such as autoencoders, kernel PCA, and t-SNE are increasingly adopted [24]. Moreover, depending on feature types, plenty of schemes have been utilized in relevant research problems. For example, PCA (Principal Component Analysis), ICA (Independent Component Analysis), and LDA (Linear Discriminant Analysis), SVD (singular value decomposition), and NMF are widely used tools which are considered under linear methods. Similarly, nonlinear methods such as kernel PCA, t-sne, MDS, isomap, autoencoder, and UMAP are also popularly used [25].

4.4 Data Balancing

In the field of reproductive medicine, several studies have explored the use of data balancing techniques to improve the accuracy and clinical utility of predictive models. For example, GhoshRoy et al. leveraged the SMOTE alongside an XGBoost classifier to predict male fertility based on clinical and lifestyle data. Their approach yielded impressive results, achieving a mean accuracy of 93.22% and an AUC of 0.98, underscoring the effectiveness of SMOTE in enhancing the recognition of the minority class, which in this case represented individuals with fertility issues. This result highlights the potential of data balancing to address class imbalance in clinical datasets, which is crucial for making reliable predictions in reproductive medicine [26]. Khodabandelu et al. [27] investigated the impact of combining SMOTE with Tomek Links and Edited Nearest Neighbours methods to balance data for predicting the success of Intrauterine Insemination (IUI). By applying these techniques, they were able to significantly reduce model bias and increase the model's sensitivity to predicting positive outcomes, such as successful IUI pregnancies. The study demonstrated that the combination of SMOTE and other data balancing methods leads to more accurate predictions that have clinical value, as it reduces the tendency for models to favour the majority class and enhances the ability to detect true positives. Kothandaraman et al. explored three different data balancing approaches such as undersampling, oversampling, and SMOTE to improve the prediction of outcomes in ART datasets. They tested these techniques across various proportions of data and found that SMOTE was the most effective method for balancing the dataset. By using SMOTE, they were able to enhance the model's ability to accurately predict positive ART outcomes, which, in turn, improved the clinical utility of the model. The results from this study provide strong evidence that balancing techniques, such as SMOTE, play a crucial role in improving predictive accuracy for ART treatments [28]. Dehghan et al. applied SMOTE oversampling to balance the IVF dataset and found that this data balancing approach led to the best performance during model training. By integrating SMOTE into the data processing phase, they were able to significantly improve the predictive power of the model, which is essential for accurately forecasting IVF success and optimizing treatment plans for patients [29]. Uyar et al. also explored various data balancing techniques, including SMOTE, undersampling, and hybrid methods, to predict successful IVF implantations. Their research demonstrated that these balancing strategies helped reduce model bias, which often favours the majority class, and enhanced the model's ability to detect true positives. When paired with evaluation metrics such as precision and the Area Under the Precision-Recall Curve (AUC-PR), these strategies produced more reliable and clinically useful predictive models. This finding underscores the importance of using the right evaluation metrics in conjunction with data balancing techniques to ensure that the predictions are both accurate and actionable [30]. GhoshRoy et al. further emphasized the value of SMOTE oversampling on highly imbalanced male fertility datasets. Their study showed that this balancing method improves the accuracy of AI models used for predicting male fertility, particularly in datasets where the number of individuals with fertility issues is significantly smaller than the number of healthy individuals. This finding is crucial because it demonstrates that even in cases of extreme class imbalance, SMOTE can effectively level the playing field, allowing the model to make more equitable and reliable predictions [31]. GhoshRoy et al. examined the effects of different data balancing methods on male fertility prediction. Their study compared various techniques, including hybrid sampling, undersampling, and oversampling, and found that hybrid sampling (a combination of oversampling and undersampling) provided the best outcomes. This approach ensured that both the minority and majority classes were well-represented in the model, leading to better predictive performance than using either oversampling or undersampling alone [32]. Yibre et al. focused on applying the SMOTE technique to male fertility data and found that it resulted in the highest accuracy when applied to the dataset. This study further supports the effectiveness of SMOTE as a tool for enhancing the performance of predictive models in fertility-related fields, where accurate predictions are critical for successful treatment outcomes [33]. Liu et al. implemented SMOTE specifically on the live birth outcome variable in their training dataset. By doing so, they were able to balance the data and reduce the risk of overfitting, a common challenge when dealing with imbalanced datasets. This application of SMOTE helped improve the robustness of their predictive model, making it more reliable in predicting live birth outcomes, which is of paramount importance in the context of IVF treatment [34].

Collectively, these studies affirm the essential role of data balancing in enabling machine learning models to uncover meaningful patterns within underrepresented clinical classes, thus supporting more equitable and accurate predictions in reproductive healthcare.

4.5 AI Tools

A diverse range of AI algorithms has been employed across key domains in reproductive medicine, including the evaluation and selection of oocytes, sperm selection and semen analysis, embryo assessment, and the prediction of IVF outcomes. The principal categories of AI methodologies applied in these areas are ML, DL, and NLP. The ML techniques are typically used to identify patterns in patient characteristics and to predict clinical outcomes by analyzing structured and multimodal datasets. In contrast, deep learning approaches are particularly well-suited for interpreting complex, high-dimensional data, such as medical imaging, time-series records, and genomic or omics data. Meanwhile, natural language processing plays a critical role in extracting clinically relevant information from unstructured data sources, most notably EHR. NLP facilitates the transformation of this unstructured text into structured, machine-readable formats, thereby enabling seamless integration with ML algorithms for further analysis. As such, NLP serves as a key enabler in leveraging the full spectrum of clinical data for AI-driven decision-making in reproductive healthcare [10, 35, 36].

AI requires access to large volumes of data and substantial computational power. The rapid advancement of graphical processing units has significantly enhanced the ability to process and analyze large-scale datasets efficiently. As hardware and software, including algorithms, continue to evolve, AI and ML are poised to significantly advance the field of reproductive medicine in the near future. Among the most widely adopted AI techniques are supervised learning algorithms, which have demonstrated notable success in various applications such as image analysis, ART outcome prediction, fertility assessment, and related areas. Table 4.1 offers a comprehensive overview of these algorithms, outlining their respective strengths and limitations. Prominent examples include decision trees, SVM, naïve Bayes, random forests, artificial neural networks, KNN, XGB, and CNNs. Their specific use cases and applications are discussed in the following sections.

DT is robust algorithm commonly used for classification and prediction tasks. In reproductive medicine, DTs are frequently applied to predict outcomes of in vitro fertilization, such as the likelihood of successful implantation or live birth, based on patient demographics and clinical data [37, 38]. Clinicians often favour this algorithm due to its "white-box" nature, offering transparent and easily interpretable decision paths. Moreover, DTs can be integrated with ensemble methods such as Random Forests and boosting techniques to enhance predictive performance.

SVM is a powerful machine learning tool that performs exceptionally well in high-dimensional spaces and complex classification problems. In reproductive medicine, SVMs have proven effective in assessing embryo quality by distinguishing between viable and non-viable embryos through analysis of morphological features [38–40]. These algorithms also support male fertility evaluation by analyzing multimodal data to predict sperm quality based on motility and morphology, aiding in

Table 4.1 Conceptual finding of widely opted algorithms in reproductive medicine

Algorithm	Key points	Key limitations	Applications in reproductive medicine
DT	Offers clear and easily interpretable decision-making pathways	Susceptible to overfitting, especially with complex datasets	Used for cost-effective decision support in elective oocyte cryopreservation and embryo transfer
SVM	Effectively handles nonlinear data with low error rates	Complex to train and difficult to interpret	Applied in sperm cell classification and embryo selection
NB	Provides rapid and accurate predictions	Assumes independence between input features, which may not hold in real-world scenarios	Utilized for predicting implantation outcomes based on embryo characteristics
RF	Addresses overfitting issues seen in decision trees; provides higher accuracy	Requires significant computational resources and ongoing maintenance	Commonly used to predict outcomes of IVF and ICSI procedures
ANNs	Easy to train and adapt; performs well even with limited training data	Requires large datasets for high predictive performance	Used for constructing predictive models for ART outcomes
XGB	Delivers high prediction accuracy; includes automatic feature selection	Operates as a black-box model; prone to overfitting with small datasets	Employed in ART success prediction, embryo selection, OHSS risk estimation, and screening for PCOS and endometriosis
CNNs	Highly effective for image analysis; rapidly advancing in medical imaging	Demands substantial computational power; limited transparency and interpretability	Applied to IVF success prediction using embryo imaging data
LR	Simple and transparent model; easy to interpret	Performs poorly with nonlinear relationships or high-dimensional datasets	Used for predicting IVF outcomes and for PCOS screening

sperm selection for intracytoplasmic sperm injection (ICSI) procedures. Additionally, SVMs contribute to comprehensive embryo viability assessments, offering valuable predictive insights that enhance IVF treatment efficacy [41, 42]. Their ability to model intricate, nonlinear relationships makes them particularly valuable in clinical contexts.

NB classifiers are among the simplest yet most effective classification algorithms, known for their reliability in medical applications. Their transparency and ease of interpretation make them especially attractive in clinical settings [43]. In IVF, NB models are employed to predict embryo implantation outcomes and assess implantation potential [44]. However, their performance may decline when input features are irrelevant, redundant, or statistically dependent [45]. To overcome these limitations, advanced variations such as semi-Naive Bayes, tree-augmented Naive Bayes, and k-dependence Bayesian classifiers have been developed to provide more robust modelling capabilities in reproductive medicine.

RF is ensemble learning methods that enhance predictive accuracy and mitigates overfitting. They are versatile and widely used in reproductive medicine for tasks such as predicting ART outcomes, evaluating embryo morphology, detecting male fertility issues, optimizing ovarian stimulation protocols, and identifying conditions like PCOS and endometriosis [46]. RFs often outperform traditional machine learning models, particularly when dealing with small datasets [47].

ANNs are extensively applied in reproductive medicine, particularly in image analysis and semen parameter prediction. They are also used to forecast IVF outcomes. The first ANN model for pregnancy prediction was introduced in 1997 [48]. Feedforward ANNs and MLPs are particularly valuable when modelling nonlinear relationships in complex datasets [49]. ANNs also support endometrial receptivity analysis, aiding in the identification of optimal embryo transfer windows to enhance implantation rates.

XGB is a high-performance gradient boosting algorithm known for its predictive accuracy and computational efficiency. In reproductive medicine, it is used for IVF outcome prediction, fertility diagnostics, and embryo classification [50]. XGB performs well across various data types, including multimodal clinical records, complex biological indicators, and time-lapse imaging. Its ability to rank feature importance provides clinicians with interpretable insights—for example, identifying key predictors such as endometrial thickness or specific genetic markers associated with pregnancy success [51].

CNNs are the most widely used deep learning models for high-dimensional data analysis, especially medical imaging. Although their "black-box" nature limits clinical transparency, CNNs have demonstrated promising applications in reproductive medicine, including sperm morphology classification, embryo quality assessment, ovarian follicle segmentation, automated fetal echocardiography, and endometrial receptivity analysis [52, 53]. CNNs excel at extracting relevant features from complex visual inputs, often outperforming traditional image-based methods. However, their widespread adoption in clinical practice remains limited by challenges related to interpretability and the need for large, annotated datasets.

LR remains a foundational tool in both statistical analysis and machine learning. It is widely employed in reproductive medicine to predict IVF success, evaluate OHSS risk, diagnose male fertility issues, and detect PCOS and endometriosis [54, 55]. LR is favoured for its simplicity, interpretability, computational efficiency, and ability to produce probabilistic outputs, making it especially valuable in clinical decision-making. Despite the rise of more complex models, LR continues to play an essential role due to its effectiveness in small datasets and straightforward implementation in real-world healthcare environments.

4.6 Proposal 1: Male Fertility Classification Using AI Tools

This section explores how AI can be used to assess male fertility through various methods, including ML and DL. Measuring sperm quality is essential to this process, with sperm evaluation being a central focus. The section is divided into three parts: the first part describes AI tools for assessing sperm morphology, the second part discusses the role of ML and DL techniques in predicting semen quality, including motility and concentration, and the third part covers computer-based and AI-driven algorithms for semen analysis.

4.6.1 Sperm Morphology Assessment

In [56], a 2001 cohort study from France with 100 participants employed the MSOME technique, reporting an AUC of 88% and finding a positive correlation with ICSI fertilization rates. A study in Iran [57], conducted in 2012, used stained sperm smear images with Bayesian classification for segmentation. It achieved accuracies of 94.3% for the sperm head, 92.4% for the acrosome, 95.1% for the nucleus, and 90.2% for the midpiece, using iterative methods based on structural similarity index and local entropy to assess sperm tail points. A 2019 study [58] analyzed 131 clinical semen samples using AI-based optical microscopy to measure sperm concentration, motility, and seminal pH, with findings strongly aligned with manual methods. Two additional studies from 2019 focused on sperm quality and morphology using the MHSMA dataset and image data [59, 60]. The first study utilized deep CNN, PCA, and KNN algorithms on low-resolution, non-stained images from the MHSMA dataset, achieving accuracies of 84.7% for acrosome, 83.9% for head, and 94.6% for vacuole, with processing speeds seven times faster than SMA and a quality grade of 95%. The second experiment applied CNN and SVM classifiers, surpassing previous work in segmenting the head, acrosome, and nucleus, achieving a dice similarity score of 0.90 for the head segment and 0.77 for the axial filament, with a quality grade of 100%. In [61], a 2020 Indian experimental study evaluated 10,163 sperm cells under stress using partially spatially coherent digital holography and quantitative phase imaging. Data inputted into seven feed-forward DNNs showed average sensitivity, specificity, and accuracy rates of 85.5%, 94.8%, and 85.6%, respectively, supporting ICSI procedures in ART. Study [62] used DMTL and DTLA algorithms on non-stained grayscale sperm images to automate abnormality detection, achieving 93.75% accuracy for vacuole identification and a quality grade of 100%. In [63], CNN models with decision-level fusion techniques were applied to datasets of both normal and abnormal sperm morphology images, achieving high classification accuracies of over 94% across three different datasets for prospective azoospermic patients, with a quality grade of 68%. In [64], a two-stage fine-tuned DNN was employed on SMIDS, HuSHeM, and SCIAN morpho datasets, reporting accuracies of 90.9%, 88.9%, and 72.1%, respectively. The fusion of deep networks improved accuracy up to 92.1%, boosting precision. Study [65] employed sparse optical flow with Lucas-Kanade and Crocker-Grier algorithms (MLP, RNN, CNN) on semen analysis and patient data, reducing the MAE from 8.83 to 7.31 in sperm motility prediction, with a quality grade of 90%. In [66], genetic neural architecture search methods with weighting factors and crossover operations were tested on the MHSMA dataset, achieving 91.7% accuracy in vacuole detection and 77.7% in acrosome detection, with a quality grade of 91%. Study [67] compared deep resolution2 (DNN), UNet4S, k-CNN, and U-Net4R techniques on GC–MS data files, reporting an AUC of 0.99. Deep resolution2 excelled in peak identification and quantification with a quality grade of 68%. In [68], a CNN-based U-Net architecture achieved a precision of 84.0% and sensitivity of 72.7% in identifying individual sperm cells, with a quality grade of 70%. In [69], algorithms including SMOreg, ML, RF, SGB, LASSO, Ridge, and XGB were evaluated on 85 videos of human semen samples and participant data. The study noted that two-stream NNs did not significantly outperform the baseline model, and participant data did not enhance predictive performance, with a quality grade of 90%. In [70], a YOLOv5 deep learning object detection technique was applied to 12 sperm specimen videos, achieving 95% accuracy across all videos and receiving a quality grade of 100%. In [71], with a quality grade of 91%, algorithms such as LR, RF, and SVM were applied to metabolomics and proteomics data using CASA and DFI datasets. Each algorithm achieved an accuracy of 87%, and differential biomarkers related to energy metabolism and oxidative stress were identified. In [72], a BPNN algorithm applied to seminal fluid data showed strong correlations between estimated and predicted values, with MAEs of 0.025, – 0.080, 0.166, and – 0.057 for protein, fructose, glucosidase, and zinc, respectively, with zinc prediction highlighted as valuable in semen analysis. In [73], a DL algorithm was applied to the JSD dataset, yielding sensitivities of 0.881 and 0.794 for abnormal and normal sperm, respectively. Study [74] applied DL, U-Net, and Mask-RCNN on the SCIAN dataset, reporting dice coefficients with transfer learning for head (0.96), acrosome (0.94), and nucleus (0.95). In [75], DL and holostain techniques were used on semen samples, achieving a structural similarity of 0.85 ± 0.03 for sperm morphology detection. In [76], the CNN algorithm was implemented on the VISEM dataset, reporting an accuracy of 91.77% for sperm head detection. Study [60] employed the SVM algorithm on semen samples, achieving an accuracy of 89.93%. In [77], SVM and CNN were used on the SCIAN dataset, with dice coefficients reported as follows: head (0.90), axial filament (0.77), acrosome (0.77), nucleus (0.78), tail (0.75), and midpiece (0.64). In [41], the HuSHem and SCIAN datasets were used to implement two DL methods, Deep CNN and VGG16, yielding true positive rates of 94.1% and 62% for the HuSHeM and SCIAN datasets, respectively. In [78], dictionary learning was applied to the SCIAN and HuSHeM datasets, with detection accuracies of 92% and 62% for the HuSHeM and SCIAN datasets, respectively. In [79], the Tail Point algorithm was applied to semen samples, reporting dice coefficient accuracies of 92% for the head, 84% for the acrosome, 87% for the nucleus, and 96% for the tail. In [80], BPNN and RBFN models were compared, with the BPNN model showing lower MAEs (0.025, – 0.080, 0.166, – 0.057) than the RBFN model based on semen samples, with a reported quality grade of 90%.

4.6.2 Semen Quality Prediction

In [81], a cross-sectional study conducted in the USA with 100 volunteers evaluated seminal quality using AI tools, including DT, MLP, and SVM. The MLP model achieved the highest predictive accuracy at 86%, outperforming the other models. In [82], a laboratory experiment involving four AI tools—MLP, SVM, Naive Bayes (NB), and DT—found that an optimized MLP model achieved the best performance with an accuracy of 93.3%. In [83], a prospective study conducted in Spain on 123 samples used MLP to assess seminal quality, obtaining accuracies of 90% for sperm concentration and 82% for motility. In [84], a laboratory experiment in Tehran compared NB, Logistic Regression, and Fuzzy C-Means, with NB achieving the highest AUC at 0.779. In [85], a study conducted in the USA implemented a Fuzzy Radial Basis Functional Neural Network, reaching a 90% accuracy rate and surpassing other classifiers, including MLP, SVM, and DT. In [86], a laboratory experiment in Zambia involving 100 volunteers used NB and ANN, with NB achieving a training accuracy of 97%. In [87], a novel approach that combined a sperm whale optimization algorithm with ANN reached an accuracy of 99.96%, outperforming existing algorithms. In [88], a laboratory experiment in China used the ESLSMOTE method to generate synthetic data, with a Back Propagation Neural Network showing the best performance and a ROC rating of 97.2%, surpassing models such as Adaptive Boosting and SVM. In [26], an Indian experiment designed a prediction model using the XGB algorithm, which achieved the highest AUC of 0.98 when compared to SVM, ADA, RF, and ET. In [31], seven ML algorithms (SVM, RF, DT, LR, NB, ADA, and MLP) were tested on a UCI dataset. The study found that DT and RF performed well, while SVM and NB had lower predictive accuracy, with RF achieving 96.7%. In [89], LASSO, Boruta, SVM-RFE, and RF were applied to transcriptome sequencing and immunohistochemical staining data, with RF achieving an AUC of 1.0 and an F-measure of 1.0. Additionally, an RF model based on transcription factors ETV2, TBX2, and ZNF689 was developed to diagnose non-obstructive azoospermia, attaining a quality grade of 74%. In [90], ANN, LASSO, SVM-RFE, LR, and RF were used on RNA-binding protein-related genes, testicular samples, clinical samples, and scENA sequencing data, achieving 74.1% accuracy on the GSE9210 cohort, 90.3% on GSE45885, 85.3% on GSE45887, and 59.1% on a local cohort. In [91], ANN and LR were applied to data on patient age, infertility duration, serum hormone levels, and testicular volumes, with ANN achieving 80% accuracy and LR 66%. The ANN model correctly predicted outcomes for 59 of the 73 patients in the test set. In [32], a predictive model using the LightGBM algorithm achieved 95.6% accuracy with synthetic data, while CatBoost performed well with 86.99% accuracy without synthetic data. In [92], sperm concentration in semen samples was evaluated using AI tools such as LR, SVM, and RF, achieving a predictive AUC of 0.72. In [93], FSNN and SPNN tools were applied, reporting accuracies of 86% and 93%, respectively. Study [94] employed an image recognition algorithm and conducted a comparative analysis, revealing a strong correlation between semen parameters (total sperm count and total motile sperm) as assessed by AI versus manual evaluation, with correlation values for sperm concentration at $r = 0.65$ ($p < 0.001$) and motility at $r = 0.84$ ($p < 0.001$). In [95], SVR, MLP, CNN, and RNN algorithms were applied to the VISEM dataset, with performances measured by MAE of 92.9%, 95%, 92.2%, and 98.6%, respectively. Study [96] utilized the THMA algorithm on semen samples, achieving an accuracy of 97.37% with a minimum execution time of 1.12 s. In [94], the Bemaner AI algorithm reported a correlation measure of $r = 0.90$ with $p < 0.001$. In [75], the CNN algorithm was applied to the VISEM dataset, resulting in a reported MAE of 2.92 for predicted sperm motility. Study [97] implemented the SVM algorithm on a dataset of semen samples, achieving an accuracy of 89.9%. In [98], the CNN algorithm was used to predict sperm DNA integrity, and results were compared with manual processes. This study found that the AI-based predictive model performed well, with a correlation value of $r = 0.97$ ($p < 0.001$). In [99], MobileNet CNN was applied to predict DNA fragmentation levels in live spermatozoa, reporting an accuracy of 90%. In [100], deepCNN was utilized to identify DFI values, showing a bivariate correlation between sperm cell images and DNA quality. In [101], a model trained on LR was applied to semen samples to detect SDF, achieving an accuracy of 82.7%. In [42], four AI tools, such as logistics regression, support vector machine, decision tree, and K-NN are used. Of all, KNN performed best, and 85% ROC is reported.

**Note: Quality grade is a scoring technique that is normalized to the total and expressed as a percentage. In healthcare, 60–80% are considered as good quality. This score is collected using a suitable tool.

4.6.3 Computer-Based and AI-Driven Tools

Computer- and AI-based systems are increasingly used for assessing semen quality, focusing on key parameters such as morphology, motility, and DNA integrity. CASA (Computer-Assisted Sperm Analysis) systems, known for their advanced optical technology, provide more accurate and consistent analyses of sperm samples and are commonly used for patients undergoing ART treatments. Recently, [102] described an automated, smartphone-based diagnostic assay that uses CASA technology to measure sperm concentration and motility. In [103], an ANN was employed to estimate sperm morphology, showing no significant difference in the percentage of normal forms compared to direct microscopic inspection. Using a CASA system, the automatic determination of the midpiece and tail achieved a quality grade of 80%. SpermQ is an advanced program for analyzing flagellar motion and is compatible with imaging techniques such as dark-field, epifluorescence, DIC, and phase-contrast microscopy [104, 105]. In [106], the authors developed a smartphone-based analyzer for on-site assessment of sperm concentration and motility, achieving 98% accuracy on unprocessed samples in under 5 s. This system aligns with WHO guidelines but has limitations when samples contain a high concentration of non-sperm cells. Mojo AISA, another AI-driven system, demonstrated reliable results comparable to manual methods, reducing analysis time by 50% (4 min per sample) in a study involving 64 participants over nine months [107]. Recently, a study confirmed CASA systems as a valid alternative for evaluating semen parameters in clinical practice, particularly for sperm concentration and motility [108]. Additionally, these systems improve efficiency and result reliability. In [109], the computer-assisted sperm analyzer (SQA-Vision) was used for detecting male fertility parameters. In [110], the authors reviewed CASA technology, highlighting its ability to assess sperm motion and morphology more accurately and objectively than traditional subjective evaluations.

After reviewing the above-mentioned cases, it is widely recognized that male fertility assessment has become more efficient with the implementation of AI tools. However, a lack of standardized protocols, proper training, and quality assessment in andrology laboratories remains a significant challenge, especially since these are essential for traditional manual processes. Even when manual semen analysis is performed by trained personnel following standardized protocols, uncertainty in interpreting results can persist. This issue is further compounded by shifts in WHO threshold values for abnormal semen quality over the years, often without sufficient explanation [111]. Thus, improvements in semen analysis are necessary, with reliability of results being a top priority. These reliable results serve as the basis for measuring fertility potential, underscoring that there is still considerable progress to be made in this field.

4.7 Proposal 2: Female Fertility Classification Using AI Tools

Female fertility is influenced by various factors, with primary clinical causes including PCOS, endometriosis, and uterine fibroids [112]. While these clinical conditions are crucial, other factors also play an important role in predicting female fertility. Much of the research on female fertility prediction remains unexplored, and as a result, researchers often concentrate on predicting these primary factors, leading to a wealth of literature on these topics. In contrast, there is relatively limited research on broader fertility detection specifically for women. This section is divided into two parts: the first part examines the role of AI in detecting or predicting PCOS, endometriosis, and uterine fibroids, and the second part focuses on the application of AI in general fertility prediction for women.

4.7.1 PCOS Detection/Classification/Prediction

In [113], a study conducted in Malaysia utilized ultrasound images to develop a model using a combination of Chan-Vese and Otsu's methods. The model demonstrated improved efficiency over the classic Chan-Vese method in quantitative evaluations. In [114], clinical and imaging data, including anthropometric and hormonal features, were used in a study in Bangladesh. Various models were tested, including GBT, RF, and LR. The highest accuracy of 91% was achieved by a hybrid Random Forest-Logistic Regression model. In Indonesia, study [115] showed that CNN was capable of automatic feature extraction on imaging data, with the CNN-based model achieving a perfect micro-average F1 score of 100%. Study [116] designed an AI-based model using electronic medical records, employing NLP and codified data to achieve a 9% false positive rate. In [117], Partial Least Squares Discriminant Analysis was applied to a metabolic dataset, yielding an AUC of 0.8 and suggesting involvement of pathways like amino acid, carbohydrate/lipid, purine, and pyrimidine metabolism. Study [118] used a Bayesian network on virtually generated clinical data, finding a 15.5% absolute mean error difference compared to physician scores and a significant positive correlation between features and physician scores (Pearson correlation = 0.82, $P = 0.01$). In [119], three AI models—NN-LVQ, K-NN, and SVM—were tested on imaging data, with SVM using an RBF kernel achieving the best accuracy at 82.55%. In study [120], four models (K-NN, SVM, NB, and RF) were applied to clinical data, with RF attaining the highest accuracy of 94%. Study [121] compared five classifiers (KNN, NB, SVM, DT, and LR) on clinical data, with DT achieving the best accuracy of 81%. In [122], imaging data was analyzed using Linear Discriminant Classifier, KNN, and SVM, with LDC showing the best accuracy at 93%. Study [123] tested multivariate logistic regression and a Bayesian classifier on clinical data, with the Bayesian classifier achieving 94% accuracy. In [124], an ANN model applied to proteomics data achieved a diagnostic accuracy of 100%. Study [125] evaluated Time-Point Feature Fusion Network and Self-Organizing Map on clinical data, with TPFFN reaching a higher accuracy of 97%. In [126], Probabilistic Neural Network, SVM, and Radial Basis Function classifiers were tested on imaging data, and PNN achieved 98% accuracy. Study [127] used SVM, RF, and LR classifiers on genetic data, with SVM attaining 100% accuracy using threefold cross-validation. In [128], SVM, RF, and Gaussian Mixture Model were tested on genetic data, with SVM achieving 100% accuracy. In [129], an SVM model applied to imaging data reached an accuracy of 94%. In [130], orthogonal PLS-DA was used on clinical data, yielding an AUC of 96%. Study [131] combined clinical and imaging data in an SVM classifier, achieving an accuracy of 95%. In [132], a combination of clinical and imaging datasets was tested with LR, KNN, CART, RF Classifier, NB, and SVM, with RFC performing best with 89% accuracy. Study [133] compared a watershed + object-growing AI model with the level set, boundary vector field, and fuzzy SVM methods. Study [134] tested SVM, RF, and GMM on genome-wide association data, identifying potential associations of circRNAs and their target genes with PCOS. In [135], imaging data was analyzed using a rule-based classifier and XGB, with the rule-based classifier achieving 97.6% accuracy. Study [136] used GBT and a rule-based classifier on imaging data, with the rule-based classifier achieving 98% accuracy. In [137], clinical data was evaluated with KNN, RF, XGB, and stacking classification algorithms, and KNN outperformed others with an accuracy of 88%. In [138], genetic data analyzed with RF and ANN classifiers saw ANN achieving the best result with an AUC of 73%. In [139], clinical data was tested with RF, SVM, LR, Gaussian NB, and ANN, with RF achieving the highest accuracy of 91%. Study [140] used frequent itemset mining and the Apriori algorithm, concluding that the Apriori algorithm provided superior results. In [141], imaging data was analyzed with LR, SVM, and Back Propagation Neural Network, with BPNN performing best. Study [142] used an SVM-based model with an accuracy of 90%. In [143], clustering analysis and manual image reading were combined on imaging data, with clustering analysis achieving 84% accuracy, outperforming manual methods. In [144], various AI techniques were tested on a reduced metabolic dataset, with SVM achieving 96% accuracy. Study [145] proposed a CNN-based model for PCOS-related data, achieving 85% accuracy using the watershed algorithm. Study [146] used a CNN algorithm with Gabor wavelet feature extraction, achieving an accuracy of 80.84%. Study [147] developed "PCONet," a CNN-based model compared with others, with PCONet achieving the highest accuracy of 98.12%. Study [148] proposed a DCNN model, reaching 84.81% accuracy. In [149], a fusion model using MobileNet for feature extraction achieved an accuracy of 82.46%. Study [150] examined transfer learning with AlexNet, Inception V3, ResNet50, and VGG16, finding that a hybrid model increased accuracy to 93%. In [151], an ANN model was compared to a Bayesian model, with ANN showing better performance. Study [152] developed a classification model based on ANN using normalized square similarity detection for feature extraction. Study [153] used ANN and NB classifiers for early PCOS diagnosis, with ANN achieving 100% accuracy. Study [154] tested SVM, CART, NB, RF, and LR, with RF achieving 96% accuracy. Study [138] used feature selection on seven classifiers, achieving optimal accuracy with the best model. In [130], clinical data was balanced using SMOTE, with LR achieving 90.9% accuracy. Study [155] designed an SVM-based model for automated detection, involving preprocessing, feature selection, segmentation, and classification. Study [156] combined SVM and KNN in an ensemble model, achieving the best F1-score of 98.06%. In [157], ten AI tools were tested, with SVM achieving the highest accuracy. Study [158] used six models, including LR, RF, KNN, SVM, NB, and a voting classifier, achieving optimal accuracy with subset selection and variance analysis. Study [159] implemented a multistack ensemble of 12 models, achieving 98% accuracy. Study [160] tested clinical data with six classifiers and developed an app for mental health condition assessment. In [161], eight tools were tested, with k-means achieving the highest accuracy of 98.9%. Study [162] used KNN, NN, SVM, DT, LR, and LDA on imaging data, with KNN reaching 97.6% accuracy. Study [163] used an ensemble of RF, ET, ADA, and MLP, achieving a maximum accuracy of 98.89%. In [164], XGB and CatBoost were tested with SMOTE, achieving 95% and 89% accuracy, respectively. In [165], an XGB model achieved 96.03% accuracy. Study [166] tested five techniques, with CatBoost achieving the highest accuracy at 92%. Study [167] found improved performance with mutual information for feature selection, with RF and ADA reaching 94%. In [168], a VGGNet16 CNN-based stacking ensemble model with XGB as the meta-learner achieved 99.89% accuracy. Finally, [148] reported 82.46% accuracy for a deep learning model based on MobileNet, compared with other architectures like VGG16, VGG19, and DenseNet. In [169], two models were proposed: the patient model and the provider model. The CBT method was used to develop these models and perform classification, with K-fold cross-validation applied to assess performance. Additionally, k-means clustering and PCA were utilized, and the results were compared in terms of prediction accuracy and feature importance. The prediction accuracy for the patient model ranged from 81 to 82.5%, while the provider model achieved a higher accuracy, ranging from 87.5 to 90.1%.

4.7.2 Diagnosis and Prediction of Endometriosis

Study [170] employed the LR algorithm to develop a supplementary diagnostic tool for detecting grade 3 and grade 4 endometriosis in infertile patients. This research was conducted with a limited sample size. Conversely, study [171] included 1016 infertile patients and utilized a LR model to predict the presence of any stage of endometriosis, including stages 3 and 4, prior to surgery. Neither study reported accuracy levels for their predictions. Study [172] evaluated 1396 symptomatic women to identify stage 3 and stage 4 endometriosis, with the predictive model achieving a sensitivity of 82.6%. In [173], a DL algorithm was used to detect all four stages of endometriosis in 213 patients, achieving a sensitivity of 100%. In [174], the genomeforest algorithm was applied to transcriptomics data, resulting in a sensitivity of 93.8%, and to methylomics data, achieving a sensitivity of 92.9%. Study [175] employed a RF algorithm to develop a predictive model for all four stages of endometriosis with a sample size of 59 patients; however, accuracy and sensitivity metrics were not reported. In the study [176], four AI tools namely DT, Partial Least Squares Discriminant Analysis (PLS-DA), SVM, and RF—were evaluated using transcriptomics and methylomics data. All models performed well, displaying varying levels of sensitivity. PLS-DA achieved the highest sensitivity (86.4%) for transcriptomics data, while DT stood out for methylomics data with a sensitivity of 76.2%. In [177], the margin tree classification algorithm was implemented on 148 endometrial samples, though accuracy metrics were not reported. In [178], the LR algorithm was applied to a dataset of 1126 patients for training and 100 for validation, with type of endometriosis (ovarian, superficial, or deep) specified. The model achieved a sensitivity of 95%. In [179], DT, RF, XGB, and a voting classifier were trained using data from 1126 patients, with 100 patients allocated for validation. The soft voting and XGB models demonstrated the highest sensitivity at 93%. Overall, all classifiers performed effectively, achieving sensitivities of 91% for DT and hard voting, and 92% for RF. In [180], LR was applied to a dataset of 1126 samples, with 789 used for training and 333 for validation, focusing on deep endometriosis with colorectal involvement. However, no performance metrics were reported. In [181], a study involving 297 patients undergoing ART included all four stages of endometriosis but did not report performance metrics. In [182], an LR-based AI model was developed using data from 326 patients, achieving a sensitivity of 68.6%, with the type of endometriosis specified. In [183], 94 patients' data were used to train an LR-based model focusing on deep endometriosis, which achieved a sensitivity of 66.7%. In [184], LR was applied to data from 228 patients, including 94 patients undergoing ART as part of the training set. The model reported a sensitivity of 68.6%. In [185], 178 cases involving patients with ovarian endometriomas were analyzed using a DT algorithm to develop a diagnostic model, but no performance metrics were reported. In [186], SVM and KNN were evaluated using 94 serum samples. KNN demonstrated superior sensitivity, achieving 100% compared to 87.5% for SVM. The study employed Raman spectroscopy and included samples from all four stages of endometriosis. In [187], PLS-DA was applied to 100 patient samples using mass spectrometry. The authors didn't specify their model sensitivity. In [188], 1-H-NMR spectroscopy was used on 45 samples with the PLS-DA algorithm, also achieving a sensitivity of 81.8%. In [189], quadratic discriminant analysis was used on 45 samples with nuclear magnetic resonance spectroscopy, but no performance metrics were provided. In [190], three AI tools—DT, GA, and the Quick Classifier Algorithm were applied to 122 samples, each achieving different sensitivities. The DT and Quick Classifier Algorithm used the same input data, while GA utilized different inputs, achieving a sensitivity of 90.9%. Similarly, between DT and the Quick Classifier Algorithm, DT demonstrated superior performance with a sensitivity of 90%. In [191], two algorithms, namely GA and DT, were used to build a model with data from 91 symptomatic patients. Among the two, DT performed best, achieving a reported sensitivity of 92.7% using the surface-enhanced laser desorption/ionization time-of-flight mass spectrometry method. In [192], a least squares SVM with matrix-assisted laser desorption ionization time-of-flight mass spectrometry analyzed 254 plasma samples, achieving sensitivities of 75% (minimal to mild), 98% (moderate to severe), and 88% (ultrasonography-negative endometriosis). In [193], the same AI technique was combined with proteomic surface-enhanced laser desorption ionization time-of-flight mass spectrometry on 49 endometriosis biopsies, reporting a sensitivity of 91%. In [189, 194, 195] different ANN models are implemented with various spectrometry techniques. In [196], 45 patients' data with nuclear magnetic resonance spectroscopy resulted in a sensitivity of 50%, with stages of endometriosis specified. In [194], surface-enhanced laser desorption on 39 patients achieved a sensitivity of 91.7%, considering all four stages. Similarly, in [195], the same method was applied to 66 serum samples, with the model also attaining a sensitivity of 91.7%. In [196], the ResNet (2 + 1) D technique was employed, utilizing 749 transvaginal ultrasound videos featuring the sliding sign. The proposed AI model achieved a sensitivity of 89%. In [197], seven AI tools, namely KNN, NB, NN, SVM, DT, RF, and LR, were applied to build a model based on image features. While all classifiers performed well, SVM achieved the highest sensitivity at 84%. In comparison, KNN, DT, and RF exhibited the lowest sensitivity, each at 66%. In [198], the LR algorithm was applied to a dataset of 189 samples, achieving sensitivities of 88% for

Model 1 (detecting deep endometriosis) and 88% for Model 2 (detecting unilateral endometria).

Moreover, the findings from case studies on endometriosis assessment represent a significant focus area and serve as a critical factor in analyzing human fertility.

4.7.3 Diagnosis of Uterine Fibroids

Study [199] introduced an AI model based on the DPCNN architecture, comparing its performance with other models such as VGG16, ResNet50, and Inception V3. The proposed model achieved a remarkable accuracy of 99.8% with the SGD optimizer. Study [200] developed a machine learning model using MRI parameters and the RF algorithm, reporting an AUC of 0.904. Similarly, study [201] proposed a deep learning model leveraging the ResNet algorithm with MRI images, achieving an accuracy of 98.8%. In [202], various machine learning algorithms, including KNN, SVM, RF, J48, and ZeroR, were analyzed and compared for their performance. Study [203] employed the DCNN algorithm, which achieved an average accuracy of 94.72% when combined with junior ultrasonographers. Notably, the standalone DCNN model outperformed this, achieving an accuracy of 95.24%, surpassing the performance of both junior and senior ultrasonographers. Study [204] implemented a deep learning-based model named MBF-CDNN, which attained an accuracy of 94.736%. Finally, study [205] proposed a hybrid model combining EfficientNet and YOLOv3, which achieved an average precision of 95%. In [206], a comparative study was performed with six ML algorithms such as DT, NB (Gaussian kernel), RF, KNN, GBT, and XGB. Each model attained diverse efficiency; of all, GBT outperformed with an accuracy of 77%. In [207], a model is proposed based on AR net (attention ResNet 101-U-net) and reported sensitivity is 84.43%. In [208], optimized U-net architecture was used to classify UF which provided a good result. In [209], a 3D nnU-Net model is developed for automatic uterus segment which is used in the clinical setting for objective assessment of therapeutic response to HIFU therapy. The reported dice score $= 0.95 \pm 0.05$. In [210], a technique using ICP and ReFineNet was proposed to register images and segment fibroid borders in ultrasound, achieving a dice coefficient of 0.879. In [211], the ICP method was used to fuse ultrasound and MR images, improving resolution for deep organs. The technique addresses dimensional discrepancies with multi-view integration and reduces noise in USgHIFU through a feature-based pipeline. In [212], a U-Net convolutional neural network was applied for automatic uterine segmentation on MRI, achieving a dice coefficient of 0.85 after hyperparameter optimization. In [213], an intelligent framework for image segmentation and enhancement was introduced, using MedGA for preprocessing. The Iterative Optimal Threshold Selection algorithm selects thresholds, which are then enhanced by MedGA. Pre-processed images achieved the best DSI values with minimal segmentation differences. In [214], a direct region detection method was employed to address MRgFUS post-treatment segmentation challenges and segment fibroids in MR images. The split-and-merge technique segmented fibroids with varying pixel intensities, validated using area and distance criteria. In [215], a fully autonomous method for segmenting the uterus and fibroids was proposed, using Iterative Optimal Threshold selection and Fuzzy C-Means clustering, with evaluation based on area and distance criteria. In [216], a three-stage segmentation network was developed to segment fibroids, employing a classification network to select fibroid slices and removing unrelated regions for final segmentation. In [217], an Inception-V4-based CNN model with transfer learning extracted features from uterine fibroid images, which were classified using an SVM, achieving 81.05% accuracy. Future improvements could include using CNN architectures like U-Net and V-Net. In [218], a hybrid CNN-transformer network identified uterine fibroids in hysteroscopy images, achieving 88.93% accuracy. In [219], a VGGNet-16 model classified endometrial lesions from hysteroscopy images with an accuracy of 80.8%. In [220], a neural network with wavelet features detected uterine fibroids, achieving 95.1% accuracy using a feedforward backpropagation neural network. In [221], a scalable EfficientNet model combined with CNN for feature extraction achieved an average accuracy of 98.88%. In [222], a DCNN model was introduced that extracted features from ultrasound images through a combination of convolutional and pooling layers. The model demonstrated an accuracy of 96.7%. In [220], a feed-forward backpropagation neural network classifier is used on ultrasonic images. The classifier achieved an accuracy of 95.1%.

The current state of research indicates that computer-aided diagnosis for UF detection has received limited attention. Existing studies primarily focus on segmentation and basic classification techniques. While many researchers have explored conditions such as uterine sarcoma and adenomyosis, both linked to infertility, these conditions are not directly related to fibroids. In contrast, UF is a leading cause of female infertility. This highlights the importance of UF detection as a promising area of research, particularly for specialists in reproductive medicine.

In [223], three AI tools namely NB, DT, and MLP were used on a limited dataset with 14 features. The three models achieved different accuracies and AUC values. Among them, DT and MLP attained the same accuracy of 74.359%, while NB achieved an accuracy of 71.795%. In [224], four classification algorithms including LDA, classification tree, RF, and bagging were applied to a larger dataset with 26 features. The authors compared the performance of these classifiers and reported an accuracy of 88% using RF. In [225], three AI models were implemented on 146 samples with 16 features. These models developed using NB, J48, and bagging classifiers, achieved varying accuracies, with the highest accuracy of 85.03% reported for the bagging classifier.

Moreover, this study identified only three articles in which researchers specifically addressed female fertility analysis. Notably, these studies did not make their data publicly available, potentially contributing to the limited research on female infertility. Consequently, this remains a highly significant and underexplored area of research within the field of reproductive medicine.

4.8 The Conceptual Overview of Case Studies

The case studies offer key insights into how AI enhances infertility assessments, surpassing traditional manual methods in efficiency and precision. Foundational AI steps, such as feature selection, extraction, and algorithm choice, have demonstrated a transformative impact on healthcare. By integrating research with clinical expertise, AI streamlines diagnostics and enables personalized infertility treatments, with a focus on reproductive science and human fertility. This section explores evolving AI techniques and their challenges, emphasizing data, algorithm choice, feature importance, and validation in reproductive medicine.

To effectively address these challenges, it is essential to curate diverse, high-quality datasets while ensuring ethical and legal considerations are met. Data plays a critical role in AI model performance, and limited data availability in fertility research remains a major issue. Fertility data is highly sensitive, often met with reluctance to share due to social stigma, cultural factors, and privacy concerns. Weak data protection laws in some regions further heighten fears of misuse for purposes beyond healthcare, such as marketing. These factors hinder trust and limit the development of robust AI models in reproductive health.

Addressing these barriers requires strong data protection laws, transparency about data usage, and public education on the benefits of data sharing for advancing healthcare. Strategies to build high-quality datasets include collaborations with hospitals, cohort studies, fertility app partnerships, voluntary data-sharing initiatives, and incentives like free health checkups. By combining these approaches and adhering to ethical standards, it is possible to curate diverse, high-quality fertility datasets while respecting privacy and consent.

Current datasets for male fertility assessments often rely on limited sample sizes, typically ranging from 100 to 131. These datasets include sperm morphology, semen analysis, sperm videos, and environmental or lifestyle factors. For female fertility, datasets are more diverse, encompassing transcriptomics, genomics, endometriosis history, ovarian reserve, ultrasound images, and clinical and genetic data related to conditions like PCOS and fibroids. Integrating these diverse data types helps researchers address reproductive health challenges and advance fertility assessments and treatments.

Feature selection techniques are pivotal in managing complex datasets. Common methods include filtering techniques, Principal Component Analysis, Pearson correlation, pretrained Convolutional Neural Networks, Recursive Feature Elimination, and ranking algorithms. These approaches reduce overfitting, mitigate bias, lower computational costs, and enhance model robustness. However, many feature selection tools remain underutilized due to resource limitations and specific research objectives. Future efforts should focus on hybrid and ensemble methods to improve performance across various datasets.

In fertility research, both conventional and advanced algorithms are employed. Traditional methods include Logistic Regression, Support Vector Machines, Random

Forest, and Decision Trees. Advanced techniques include XGBoost, Deep Multi-task Learning (DMTL), Convolutional Neural Networks, and Genetic Algorithms. Reported accuracies range from 66 to 98%, with AUC values from 80 to 100%, underscoring the efficacy of these methods in binary classification tasks commonly used in fertility analysis.

Advances like Computer-Aided Sperm Analysis further illustrate AI's potential to improve accuracy and reduce variability in fertility assessments. ML and DL approaches show strong predictive capabilities, offering precise and reliable outcomes. These advancements highlight the transformative impact of AI in fertility research and clinical practice, paving the way for innovative solutions to reproductive health challenges.

Moreover, the acceptance of AI models in reproductive science remains uncertain. A significant challenge lies in ensuring data quality and accessibility, which are closely tied to ethical management. Without high-quality, diverse datasets, developing robust models is difficult. Even when models are created, validation becomes a critical step that requires external datasets. Without such data, biases can emerge, undermining the model's reliability.

Additionally, the complexity of AI models often makes it challenging for clinicians to understand their functionality and decision-making processes. This lack of understanding leads to skepticism and hesitancy in adopting AI methodologies. Clinicians are integral to medical science, and without their trust and involvement, widespread acceptance of AI models becomes a significant challenge. Bridging the gap between clinical management and AI scientists is crucial for fostering collaboration and facilitating the integration of AI into reproductive healthcare.

4.9 Conclusion

The core AI principles, including dataset preparation, feature engineering, algorithm selection, and performance evaluation, cover aspects of human fertility assessment using AI tools and their advancements, as illustrated through case studies. Notably, only a few AI-based applications have been implemented in medical practice and management. To address the main barriers, key challenges and potential solutions are thoroughly discussed. The next few decades will require more research focusing on human fertility. It is widely recognized that infertility can sometimes be treated or managed effectively, particularly when detected early. With the advancement of transformative technology, identifying infertility has become easier and more effective, greatly enhancing the chances of conception. Additionally, the highlighted evidence is clearly presented and encourages researchers to take a proactive and systematic approach to addressing critical issues in fertility research.

References

1. Dergham, A., Liblik, K., Witherspoon, L., & Flannigan, R. (2025). Reproductive medicine and AI. In *Artificial intelligence in urology* (pp. 275–294). Academic Press.
2. Hajirasouliha, I., & Elemento, O. (2020). Precision medicine and artificial intelligence: Overview and relevance to reproductive medicine. *Fertility and Sterility, 114*(5), 908–913.
3. Iftikhar, P., Kuijpers, M. V., Khayyat, A., Iftikhar, A., & De Sa, M. D. (2020). Artificial intelligence: a new paradigm in obstetrics and gynecology research and clinical practice. *Cureus, 12*(2).
4. He, J., Baxter, S. L., Xu, J., Xu, J., Zhou, X., & Zhang, K. (2019). The practical implementation of artificial intelligence technologies in medicine. *Nature Medicine, 25*(1), 30–36.
5. Devjak, R., Papler, T. B., Verdenik, I., Tacer, K. F., & Bokal, E. V. (2016). Embryo quality predictive models based on cumulus cells gene expression. *Balkan Journal of Medical Genetics: BJMG, 19*(1), 5.
6. Martin, A. R., Kanai, M., Kamatani, Y., Okada, Y., Neale, B. M., & Daly, M. J. (2019). Clinical use of current polygenic risk scores may exacerbate health disparities. *Nature Genetics, 51*(4), 584–591.
7. Shaker, F. (2018). Human sperm head morphology dataset (hushem). *Mendeley Data, 3*.
8. AACR Project Genie Consortium, AACR Project GENIE Consortium, André, F., Arnedos, M., Baras, A. S., Baselga, J., Bedard, P. L., Berger, M. F., Bierkens, M., Calvo, F., Cerami, E., Chakravarty, D., Dang, K. K., Davidson, N. E., Del Vecchio Fitz, C., Dogan, S., DuBois, R. N., Ducar, M. D., Andrew Futreal, P., et al. (2017). AACR Project GENIE: powering precision medicine through an international consortium. *Cancer Discovery, 7*(8), 818–831.
9. Patel, B. N., Rosenberg, L., Willcox, G., Baltaxe, D., Lyons, M., Irvin, J., Rajpurkar, P., Amrhein, T., Gupta, R., Halabi, S., & Langlotz, C. (2019). Human–machine partnership with artificial intelligence for chest radiograph diagnosis. *NPJ Digital Medicine, 2*(1), 111.
10. Bansod, A. R., Jha, R. K., More, A., & Fadnavis, R. A. (2022). Artificial intelligence in reproductive medicine. *Journal of Datta Meghe Institute of Medical Sciences University, 17*(2), 499–503.
11. Wdowiak, N., Wójtowicz, K., Wdowiak-Filip, A., Pucek, W., Wróbel, A., Wróbel, J., & Wdowiak, A. (2024). Environmental factors as the main hormonal disruptors of male fertility. *Journal of Clinical Medicine, 13*(7), 1986.
12. Taebi, M., & Meamar, F. Z. (2024). Healthy fertility and environmental sustainability: A narrative review. *Journal of Isfahan Medical School.*
13. Delbaere, I., Verbiest, S., & Tydén, T. (2020). Knowledge about the impact of age on fertility: A brief review. *Upsala Journal of Medical Sciences, 125*(2), 167–174.
14. ESHRE Capri Workshop Group. (2005). Fertility and ageing. *Human Reproduction Update, 11*(3), 261–276.
15. Kim, S. W., Ki, M. S., Kim, C. L., Hwang, I. S., & Jeon, I. S. (2017). A simple confocal microscopy-based method for assessing sperm movement. *Development & Reproduction, 21*(3), 229.
16. Chen, Z., Wang, Z., Du, M., & Liu, Z. (2022). Artificial intelligence in the assessment of female reproductive function using ultrasound: A review. *Journal of Ultrasound in Medicine, 41*(6), 1343–1353.
17. Aggarwal, R., Sounderajah, V., Martin, G., Ting, D. S., Karthikesalingam, A., King, D., Ashrafian, H., & Darzi, A. (2021). Diagnostic accuracy of deep learning in medical imaging: A systematic review and meta-analysis. *NPJ Digital Medicine, 4*(1), 65.
18. Wang, R., Pan, W., Jin, L., Li, Y., Geng, Y., Gao, C., Chen, G., Wang, H., Ma, D., & Liao, S. (2019). Artificial intelligence in reproductive medicine. *Reproduction, 158*(4), R139–R154.
19. Cai, J., Jiang, X., Liu, L., Liu, Z., Chen, J., Chen, K., Yang, X., & Ren, J. (2024). Pretreatment prediction for IVF outcomes: generalized applicable model or centre-specific model?. *Human Reproduction, 39*(2), 364–373.

20. Sanz, H., Valim, C., Vegas, E., Oller, J. M., & Reverter, F. (2018). SVM-RFE: Selection and visualization of the most relevant features through non-linear kernels. *BMC Bioinformatics, 19*, 1–18.
21. Zhu, S., Jiang, W., Sun, Y., Chen, L., Li, R., Chen, X., & Zheng, B. (2024). Nomogram to predict the probability of clinical pregnancy in women with poor ovarian response undergoing in vitro fertilization/intracytoplasmic sperm injection cycles. *Archives of Gynecology and Obstetrics, 310*(3), 1697–1707.
22. Zad, Z., Jiang, V. S., Wolf, A. T., Wang, T., Cheng, J. J., Paschalidis, I. C., & Mahalingaiah, S. (2024). Predicting polycystic ovary syndrome with machine learning algorithms from electronic health records. *Frontiers in Endocrinology, 15*, 1298628.
23. Zandbaaf, S., Khorrami, M. R. K., Garmarudi, A. B., & Rashidi, B. H. (2020). Diagnosis of pregnancy-based classification of embryo culture medium samples by infrared spectrometry and chemometrics. *Infrared Physics & Technology, 104*, Article 103069.
24. Kobak, D., & Berens, P. (2019). The art of using t-SNE for single-cell transcriptomics. *Nature Communications, 10*(1), 5416.
25. Liu, K., Zhang, Y., Martin, C., Ma, X., & Shen, B. (2022). Translational bioinformatics for human reproductive biology research: Examples, opportunities and challenges for a future reproductive medicine. *International Journal of Molecular Sciences, 24*(1), 4.
26. GhoshRoy, D., Alvi, P. A., & Santosh, K. C. (2022). Explainable AI to predict male fertility using extreme gradient boosting algorithm with SMOTE. *Electronics, 12*(1), 15.
27. Khodabandelu, S., Basirat, Z., Khaleghi, S., Khafri, S., Montazery Kordy, H., & Golsorkhtabaramiri, M. (2022). Developing machine learning-based models to predict intrauterine insemination (IUI) success by address modeling challenges in imbalanced data and providing modification solutions for them. *BMC Medical Informatics and Decision Making, 22*(1), 228.
28. Kothandaraman, R., Andavar, S., & Raj, R. S. P. (2021). Dynamic model for assisted reproductive technology outcome prediction. *Brazilian Archives of Biology and Technology, 64*, Article e21200758.
29. Dehghan, S., Rabiei, R., Choobineh, H., Maghooli, K., Nazari, M., & Vahidi-Asl, M. (2024). Comparative study of machine learning approaches integrated with genetic algorithm for IVF success prediction. *PLoS ONE, 19*(10), Article e0310829.
30. Uyar, A., Bener, A., Ciracy, H. N., & Bahceci, M. (2010). Handling the imbalance problem of IVF implantation prediction. *IAENG International Journal of Computer Science, 37*(2), 164–170.
31. GhoshRoy, D., Alvi, P. A., & Santosh, K. C. (2023, March). Unboxing industry-standard AI models for male fertility prediction with SHAP. In *Healthcare* (Vol. 11, No. 7, p. 929). MDPI.
32. GhoshRoy, D., Alvi, P. A., & Santosh, K. C. (2024). Leveraging sampling schemes on skewed class distribution to enhance male fertility detection with ensemble AI learners. *International Journal of Pattern Recognition and Artificial Intelligence, 38*(02), 2451003.
33. Yibre, A. M., & Koçer, B. (2021). Semen quality predictive model using feed forwarded neural network trained by learning-based artificial algae algorithm. *Engineering Science and Technology, an International Journal, 24*(2), 310–318.
34. Liu, L., Liu, B., Liao, M., Gan, Q., Huang, Q., & Yang, Y. (2024). Identifying key predictive features for live birth rate in advanced maternal age patients undergoing single vitrified-warmed blastocyst transfer. *Reproductive Biology and Endocrinology, 22*(1), 120.
35. Curchoe, C. L., Farias, A. F. S., Mendizabal-Ruiz, G., & Chavez-Badiola, A. (2020). Evaluating predictive models in reproductive medicine. *Fertility and Sterility, 114*(5), 921–926.
36. Luong, T. M. T., & Le, N. Q. K. (2024). Artificial intelligence in time-lapse system: Advances, applications, and future perspectives in reproductive medicine. *Journal of Assisted Reproduction and Genetics, 41*(2), 239–252.
37. Carrasco, B., Arroyo, G., Gil, Y., Gómez, M. J., Rodríguez, I., Barri, P. N., Veiga, A., & Boada, M. (2017). Selecting embryos with the highest implantation potential using data mining and decision tree based on classical embryo morphology and morphokinetics. *Journal of Assisted Reproduction and Genetics, 34*, 983–990.

38. Mesen, T. B., Mersereau, J. E., Kane, J. B., & Steiner, A. Z. (2015). Optimal timing for elective egg freezing. *Fertility and Sterility, 103*(6), 1551–1556.
39. Lee, R. K. K., Hou, J. W., Ho, H. Y., Hwu, Y. M., Lin, M. H., Tsai, Y. C., & Su, J. T. (2002). Sperm morphology analysis using strict criteria as a prognostic factor in intrauterine insemination. *International journal of andrology, 25*(5), 277–280.
40. Tseng, K. K., Li, Y., Hsu, C. Y., Huang, H. N., Zhao, M., & Ding, M. (2013). Computer-assisted system with multiple feature fused support vector machine for sperm morphology diagnosis. *BioMed Research International, 2013*(1), Article 687607.
41. Mirsky, S. K., Barnea, I., Levi, M., Greenspan, H., & Shaked, N. T. (2017). Automated analysis of individual sperm cells using stain-free interferometric phase microscopy and machine learning. *Cytometry Part A, 91*(9), 893–900.
42. Roy, D. G., & Alvi, P. A. (2021, December). Detection of male fertility using AI-driven tools. In *International Conference on Recent Trends in Image Processing and Pattern Recognition* (pp. 14–25). Springer International Publishing.
43. Morales, D. A., Bengoetxea, E., Larrañaga, P., García, M., Franco, Y., Fresnada, M., & Merino, M. (2008). Bayesian classification for the selection of in vitro human embryos using morphological and clinical data. *Computer Methods and Programs in Biomedicine, 90*(2), 104–116.
44. Langley, P., & Sage, S. (1994, January). Induction of selective Bayesian classifiers. In *Uncertainty in Artificial Intelligence* (pp. 399–406). Morgan Kaufmann.
45. Pazzani, M. J. (1995, January). Searching for dependencies in Bayesian classifiers. In *Pre-proceedings of the Fifth International Workshop on Artificial Intelligence and Statistics* (pp. 424–429). PMLR.
46. Hassan, M. R., Al-Insaif, S., Hossain, M. I., & Kamruzzaman, J. (2020). A machine learning approach for prediction of pregnancy outcome following IVF treatment. *Neural Computing and Applications, 32*(7), 2283–2297.
47. Romano, A., Rižner, T. L., Werner, H. M. J., Semczuk, A., Lowy, C., Schröder, C., Griesbeck, A., Adamski, J., Fishman, D., & Tokarz, J. (2023). Endometrial cancer diagnostic and prognostic algorithms based on proteomics, metabolomics, and clinical data: A systematic review. *Frontiers in Oncology, 13*, 1120178.
48. Wołczyński, S., Szamatowicz, J., Milewska, A. J., Domitrz, J., Jamiołkowski, J., & Milewski, R. (2009). Prognosis of the IVF ICSI/ET procedure efficiency with the use of artificial neural networks among patients of the Department of Reproduction and Gynecological Endocrinology. *Ginekologia Polska, 80*(12).
49. Cavalera, F., Zanoni, M., Merico, V., Bui, T. T. H., Belli, M., Fassina, L., Garagna, S., & Zuccotti, M. (2018). A neural network-based identification of developmentally competent or incompetent mouse fully-grown oocytes. *Journal of Visualized Experiments: JoVE*, (133), 56668.
50. Li, Y., Duan, H., & Wang, S. (2023). An XGBoost predictive model of ongoing pregnancy in patients following hysteroscopic adhesiolysis. *Reproductive BioMedicine Online, 46*(6), 965–972.
51. Li, X., Ono, C., Warita, N., Shoji, T., Nakagawa, T., Usukura, H., et al. (2022). Heart rate information-based machine learning prediction of emotions among pregnant women. *Frontiers in Psychiatry, 12*, 799029.
52. Karthik, Y., Sruthi, R., & Sujithra, M. (2024, October). Polycystic Ovary Syndrome Prediction through CNN based Image Analysis: A Deep Learning Based Approach. In *2024 8th International Conference on I-SMAC (IoT in Social, Mobile, Analytics and Cloud)(I-SMAC)* (pp. 1547–1553). IEEE.
53. Chai, R., & Gunawan, D. (2022). Optimizing CNN hyperparameters for blastocyst quality assessment in small datasets. *IEEE Access, 10*, 88621–88631.
54. Zhao, X., Liu, Y., Zhang, A., Gao, B., Feng, Q., Huang, H., Zhu, X., Sun, X., & Xu, D. (2020). Logistic regression analyses of factors affecting fertility of intrauterine adhesions patients. *Annals of Translational Medicine, 8*(4), 49.

55. Lin, J., & Sun, X. X. (2018). Predictive modeling in reproductive medicine. *Reproductive and Developmental Medicine, 2*(04), 224–229.
56. Bartoov, B., Berkovitz, A., Eltes, F., Kogosowski, A., Menezo, Y., & Barak, Y. (2002). Real-time fine morphology of motile human sperm cells is associated with IVF-ICSI outcome. *Journal of Andrology, 23*(1), 1–8.
57. Bijar, A., Mikaeili, M., & Khayati, R. (2012). Fully automatic identification and discrimination of sperm's parts in microscopic images of stained human semen smear. *Journal of Biomedical Science and Engineering, 5*(2012).
58. Agarwal, A., Henkel, R., Huang, C. C., & Lee, M. S. (2019). Automation of human semen analysis using a novel artificial intelligence optical microscopic technology. *Andrologia, 51*(11), Article e13440.
59. Javadi, S., & Mirroshandel, S. A. (2019). A novel deep learning method for automatic assessment of human sperm images. *Computers in Biology and Medicine, 109*, 182–194.
60. Movahed, R. A., Mohammadi, E., & Orooji, M. (2019). Automatic segmentation of Sperm's parts in microscopic images of human semen smears using concatenated learning approaches. *Computers in Biology and Medicine, 109*, 242–253.
61. Butola, A., Popova, D., Prasad, D. K., Ahmad, A., Habib, A., Tinguely, J. C., Basnet, P., Acharya, G., Senthilkumaran, P., Mehta, D.S., & Ahluwalia, B. S. (2020). High spatially sensitive quantitative phase imaging assisted with deep neural network for classification of human spermatozoa under stressed condition. *Scientific Reports, 10*(1), 13118.
62. Abbasi, A., Miahi, E., & Mirroshandel, S. A. (2021). Effect of deep transfer and multi-task learning on sperm abnormality detection. *Computers in Biology and Medicine, 128*, Article 104121.
63. Yüzkat, M., Ilhan, H. O., & Aydin, N. (2021). Multi-model CNN fusion for sperm morphology analysis. *Computers in Biology and Medicine, 137*, Article 104790.
64. Ilhan, H. O., & Serbes, G. (2022). Sperm morphology analysis by using the fusion of two-stage fine-tuned deep networks. *Biomedical Signal Processing and Control, 71*, Article 103246.
65. Ottl, S., Amiriparian, S., Gerczuk, M., & Schuller, B. W. (2022). motilitAI: A machine learning framework for automatic prediction of human sperm motility. *iScience, 25*.
66. Miahi, E., Mirroshandel, S. A., & Nasr, A. (2022). Genetic neural architecture search for automatic assessment of human sperm images. *Expert Systems with Applications, 188*, Article 115937.
67. Fan, X., Xu, Z., Zhang, H., Liu, D., Yang, Q., Tao, Q., Wen, M., Kang, X., Zhang, Z., & Lu, H. (2022). Fully automatic resolution of untargeted GC-MS data with deep learning assistance. *Talanta, 244*, 123415.
68. Lee, R., Witherspoon, L., Robinson, M., Lee, J. H., Duffy, S. P., Flannigan, R., & Ma, H. (2022). Automated rare sperm identification from low-magnification microscopy images of dissociated microsurgical testicular sperm extraction samples using deep learning. *Fertility and Sterility, 118*(1), 90–99.
69. Huang, H. H., Hsieh, S. J., Chen, M. S., Jhou, M. J., Liu, T. C., Shen, H. L., Yang, C. T., Hung, C. C., Yu, Y. Y., & Lu, C. J. (2023). Machine learning predictive models for evaluating risk factors affecting sperm count: predictions based on health screening indicators. *Journal of Clinical Medicine, 12*(3), 1220.
70. Yuzkat, M., Ilhan, H. O., & Aydin, N. (2023). Detection of sperm cells by single-stage and two-stage deep object detectors. *Biomedical Signal Processing and Control, 83*, Article 104630.
71. Guo, Y., Li, J., Hao, F., Yang, Y., Yang, H., Chang, Q., Kong, P., Liu, W., Jiao, X., & Teng, X. (2023). A new perspective on semen quality of aged male: The characteristics of metabolomics and proteomics. *Frontiers in Endocrinology, 13*, 1058250.
72. Sato, T., Kishi, H., Murakata, S., Hayashi, Y., Hattori, T., Nakazawa, S., et al. (2022). A new deep-learning model using YOLOv3 to support sperm selection during intracytoplasmic sperm injection procedure. *Reproductive Medicine and Biology, 21*(1), e12454.
73. Marín, R., & Chang, V. (2021). Impact of transfer learning for human sperm segmentation using deep learning. *Computers in Biology and Medicine, 136*, Article 104687.

74. Nygate, Y. N., Levi, M., Mirsky, S. K., Turko, N. A., Rubin, M., Barnea, I., Dardikman-Yoffe, G., Haifler, M., Shalev, A., & Shaked, N. T. (2020). Holographic virtual staining of individual biological cells. *Proceedings of the National Academy of Sciences, 117*(17), 9223–9231.
75. Valiuškaitė, V., Raudonis, V., Maskeliūnas, R., Damaševičius, R., & Krilavičius, T. (2020). Deep learning-based evaluation of spermatozoid motility for artificial insemination. *Sensors, 21*(1), 72.
76. Dubey, V., Popova, D., Ahmad, A., Acharya, G., Basnet, P., Mehta, D. S., & Ahluwalia, B. S. (2019). Partially spatially coherent digital holographic microscopy and machine learning for quantitative analysis of human spermatozoa under oxidative stress condition. *Scientific Reports, 9*(1), 3564.
77. Riordon, J., McCallum, C., & Sinton, D. (2019). Deep learning for the classification of human sperm. *Computers in Biology and Medicine, 111*, Article 103342.
78. Shaker, F., Monadjemi, S. A., Alirezaie, J., & Naghsh-Nilchi, A. R. (2017). A dictionary learning approach for human sperm heads classification. *Computers in Biology and Medicine, 91*, 181–190.
79. Shaker, F., Monadjemi, S. A., & Naghsh-Nilchi, A. R. (2016). Automatic detection and segmentation of sperm head, acrosome and nucleus in microscopic images of human semen smears. *Computer Methods and Programs in Biomedicine, 132*, 11–20.
80. Vickram, A. S., Kamini, A. R., Das, R., Pathy, M. R., Parameswari, R., Archana, K., & Sridharan, T. B. (2016). Validation of artificial neural network models for predicting biochemical markers associated with male infertility. *Systems Biology in Reproductive Medicine, 62*(4), 258–265.
81. Gil, D., Girela, J. L., De Juan, J., Gomez-Torres, M. J., & Johnsson, M. (2012). Predicting seminal quality with artificial intelligence methods. *Expert Systems with Applications, 39*(16), 12564–12573.
82. Bidgoli, A. A., Komleh, H. E., & Mousavirad, S. J. (2015, November). Seminal quality prediction using optimized artificial neural network with genetic algorithm. In *2015 9th International Conference on Electrical and Electronics Engineering (ELECO)* (pp. 695–699). IEEE.
83. Girela, J. L., Gil, D., Johnsson, M., Gomez-Torres, M. J., & De Juan, J. (2013). Semen parameters can be predicted from environmental factors and lifestyle using artificial intelligence methods. *Biology of Reproduction, 88*(4), 99–101.
84. Soltanzadeh, S., Zarandi, M. H. F., & Astanjin, M. B. (2016, October). A hybrid fuzzy clustering approach for fertile and unfertile analysis. In *2016 Annual Conference of the North American Fuzzy Information Processing Society (NAFIPS)* (pp. 1–6). IEEE.
85. Candemir, C. (2018). Estimating the semen quality from life style using fuzzy radial basis functions. *International Journal of Machine Learning (IJML), 8*(1), 44–48.
86. Simfukwe, M., Kunda, D., & Chembe, C. (2015). Comparing naive bayes method and artificial neural network for semen quality categorization. *International Journal of Innovative Science and Research Technology, 2*(7), 689–694.
87. Engy, E. L., Ali, E. L., & Sally, E. G. (2018). An optimized artificial neural network approach based on sperm whale optimization algorithm for predicting fertility quality. *Studies in Informatics and Control, 27*(3), 349–358.
88. Ma, J., Afolabi, D. O., Ren, J., & Zhen, A. (2021). Predicting seminal quality via imbalanced learning with evolutionary safe-level synthetic minority over-sampling technique. *Cognitive Computation, 13*(4), 833–844.
89. Zhou, R., Liang, J., Chen, Q., Tian, H., Yang, C., & Liu, C. (2023). A 3-gene random forest model to diagnose non-obstructive azoospermia based on transcription factor-related henes. *Reproductive Sciences, 30*(1), 233–246.
90. Peng, F., Muhuitijiang, B., Zhou, J., Liang, H., Zhang, Y., & Zhou, R. (2023). An artificial neural network model to diagnose non-obstructive azoospermia based on RNA-binding protein-related genes. *Aging (Albany NY), 15*(8), 3120.
91. Samli, M. M., & Dogan, I. (2004). An artificial neural network for predicting the presence of spermatozoa in the testes of men with nonobstructive azoospermia. *The Journal of Urology, 171*(6), 2354–2357.

92. Ory, J., Tradewell, M. B., Blankstein, U., Lima, T. F., Nackeeran, S., Gonzalez, D. C., Nwefo, E., Moryousef, J., Madhusoodanan, V., Lau, S., Jarvi, K., & Ramasamy, R. (2022). Artificial intelligence-based machine learning models predict sperm parameter upgrading after varicocele repair: a multi-institutional analysis. *The World Journal of Men's Health, 40*(4), 618.
93. Lesani, A., Kazemnejad, S., Zand, M. M., Azadi, M., Jafari, H., Mofrad, M. R., & Nosrati, R. (2020). Quantification of human sperm concentration using machine learning-based spectrophotometry. *Computers in Biology and Medicine, 127*, Article 104061.
94. Tsai, V. F., Zhuang, B., Pong, Y. H., Hsieh, J. T., & Chang, H. C. (2020). Web-and artificial intelligence–based image recognition for sperm motility analysis: Verification study. *JMIR Medical Informatics, 8*(11), Article e20031.
95. Ottl, S., Amiriparian, S., Gerczuk, M., & Schuller, B. W. (2022). motilitAI: A machine learning framework for automatic prediction of human sperm motility. *iscience, 25*(8).
96. Somasundaram, D., & Nirmala, M. (2021). Faster region convolutional neural network and semen tracking algorithm for sperm analysis. *Computer Methods and Programs in Biomedicine, 200*, Article 105918.
97. Goodson, S. G., White, S., Stevans, A. M., Bhat, S., Kao, C. Y., Jaworski, S., Marlowe, T. R., Kohlmeier, M., McMillan, L., Zeisel, S. H., & O'Brien, D. A. (2017). CASAnova: A multiclass support vector machine model for the classification of human sperm motility patterns. *Biology of Reproduction*, *97*(5), 698–708.
98. Kuroda, S., Karna, K. K., Kaiyal, R. S., Cannarella, R., Lundy, S. D., Vij, S. C., & Agarwal, A. (2023). Novel sperm chromatin dispersion test with artificial intelligence-aided halo evaluation: A comparison study with existing modalities. *Andrology, 11*(8), 1581–1592.
99. Noy, L., Barnea, I., Mirsky, S. K., Kamber, D., Levi, M., & Shaked, N. T. (2023). Sperm-cell DNA fragmentation prediction using label-free quantitative phase imaging and deep learning. *Cytometry Part A, 103*(6), 470–478.
100. McCallum, C., Riordon, J., Wang, Y., Kong, T., You, J. B., Sanner, S., Lagunov, A., Hannam, T.G., Jarvi, K., & Sinton, D. (2019). Deep learning-based selection of human sperm with high DNA integrity. *Communications Biology*, *2*(1), 250.
101. Wang, Y., Riordon, J., Kong, T., Xu, Y., Nguyen, B., Zhong, J., You, J. B., Lagunov, A., Hannam, T. G., Jarvi, K., & Sinton, D. (2019). Prediction of DNA integrity from morphological parameters using a single-sperm DNA fragmentation index assay. *Advanced Science*, *6*(15), 1900712.
102. Steigerwald, P., & Krause, W. (1998). Estimation of sperm morphology using a new GASA system. *Andrologia, 30*(1), 23–27.
103. AS, V., Das, R., MS, S., Rao, K. A., & TB, S. (2013). Prediction of Zn concentration in human seminal plasma of Normospermia samples by Artificial Neural Networks (ANN). *Journal of Assisted Reproduction and Genetics, 30*, 453–459.
104. Hansen, J. N., Rassmann, S., Jikeli, J. F., & Wachten, D. (2018). SpermQ–a simple analysis software to comprehensively study flagellar beating and sperm steering. *Cells, 8*(1), 10.
105. Wachten, D., Jikeli, J. F., & Kaupp, U. B. (2017). Sperm sensory signaling. *Cold Spring Harbor Perspectives in Biology, 9*(7), Article a028225.
106. Kanakasabapathy, M. K., Sadasivam, M., Singh, A., Preston, C., Thirumalaraju, P., Venkataraman, M., Bormann, C. L., Draz, M. S., Petrozza, J. C., & Shafiee, H. (2017). An automated smartphone-based diagnostic assay for point-of-care semen analysis. *Science Translational Medicine*, *9*(382), eaai7863.
107. Sengupta, P., Dutta, S., Roychoudhury, S., Vizzarri, F., & Slama, P. (2023). Revolutionizing semen analysis: Introducing Mojo AISA, the next-gen artificial intelligence microscopy. *Frontiers in Cell and Developmental Biology, 11*, 1203708.
108. Finelli, R., Leisegang, K., Tumallapalli, S., Henkel, R., & Agarwal, A. (2021). The validity and reliability of computer-aided semen analyzers in performing semen analysis: A systematic review. *Translational Andrology and Urology, 10*(7), 3069.
109. Agarwal, A., Selvam, M. K. P., Sharma, R., Master, K., Sharma, A., Gupta, S., & Henkel, R. (2018). Home sperm testing device versus laboratory sperm quality analyzer: Comparison of motile sperm concentration. *Fertility and sterility, 110*(7), 1277–1284.

110. Singh, A. K., Kumar, A., & Bisla, A. (2021). Computer-assisted sperm analysis (CASA) in veterinary science: A review. *The Indian Journal of Animal Sciences, 91*(6), 419–429.
111. Barbieri, R. L. (2019). Female infertility. In *Yen and Jaffe's reproductive endocrinology* (pp. 556–581). Elsevier
112. Nazarudin, A. A., Zulkarnain, N., Mokri, S. S., Zaki, W. M. D. W., & Hussain, A. (2020, November). An implementation of Otsu thresholding and the Chan–Vese method on the PCO segmentation of ultrasound images. In *2020 2nd International Conference on Electrical, Control and Instrumentation Engineering (ICECIE)* (pp. 1–9). IEEE.
113. Bharati, S., Podder, P., & Mondal, M. R. H. (2020, June). Diagnosis of polycystic ovary syndrome using machine learning algorithms. In *2020 IEEE Region 10 Symposium (TENSYMP)* (pp. 1486–1489). IEEE.
114. Cahyono, B., Mubarok, M. S., & Wisesty, U. N. (2017, May). An implementation of convolutional neural network on PCO classification based on ultrasound image. In *2017 5th International Conference on Information and Communication Technology (ICoIC7)* (pp. 1–4). IEEE.
115. Castro, V., Shen, Y., Yu, S., Finan, S., Pau, C. T., Gainer, V., Keefe, C.C., Savova, G., Murphy, S.N., Cai, T., & Welt, C. K. (2015). Identification of subjects with polycystic ovary syndrome using electronic health records. *Reproductive Biology and Endocrinology, 13*, 1-8.
116. RoyChoudhury, S., Mishra, B. P., Khan, T., Chattopadhayay, R., Lodh, I., Ray, C. D., Bose, G., Sarkar, H. S., Srivastava, S., Joshi, M. V., Chakravarty, B., & Chaudhury, K. (2016). Serum metabolomics of Indian women with polycystic ovary syndrome using 1 H NMR coupled with a pattern recognition approach. *Molecular BioSystems, 12*(11), 3407–3416.
117. Rodriguez, E. M., Thomas, D., Druet, A., Vlajic-Wheeler, M., Lane, K. J., & Mahalingaiah, S. (2020). Identifying women at risk for polycystic ovary syndrome using a mobile health app: Virtual tool functionality assessment. *JMIR Formative Research, 4*(5), Article e15094.
118. Purnama, B., Wisesti, U. N., Nhita, F., Gayatri, A., & Mutiah, T. (2015, May). A classification of polycystic Ovary Syndrome based on follicle detection of ultrasound images. In *2015 3rd international conference on information and communication technology (ICoICT)* (pp. 396–401). IEEE.
119. Prapty, A. S., & Shitu, T. T. (2020, December). An efficient decision tree establishment and performance analysis with different machine learning approaches on polycystic ovary syndrome. In *2020 23rd international conference on computer and information technology (ICCIT)* (pp. 1–5). IEEE.
120. Chauhan, P., Patil, P., Rane, N., Raundale, P., & Kanakia, H. (2021, June). Comparative analysis of machine learning algorithms for prediction of pcos. In *2021 international conference on communication information and computing technology (ICCICT)* (pp. 1–7). IEEE.
121. Lawrence, M. J., Eramian, M. G., Pierson, R. A., & Neufeld, E. (2007, May). Computer assisted detection of polycystic ovary morphology in ultrasound images. In *Fourth Canadian Conference on Computer and Robot Vision (CRV'07)* (pp. 105–112). IEEE.
122. Mehrotra, P., Chatterjee, J., Chakraborty, C., Ghoshdastidar, B., & Ghoshdastidar, S. (2011, December). Automated screening of polycystic ovary syndrome using machine learning techniques. In *2011 Annual IEEE India conference* (pp. 1–5). IEEE.
123. Matharoo-Ball, B., Hughes, C., Lancashire, L., Tooth, D., Ball, G., Creaser, C., Elgasim, M., Rees, R., Layfield, R., & Atiomo, W. (2007). Characterization of biomarkers in polycystic ovary syndrome (PCOS) using multiple distinct proteomic platforms. *Journal of Proteome Research, 6*(8), 3321–3328.
124. Lehtinen, J. C., Forsström, J., Koskinen, P., Penttilä, T. A., Järvi, T., & Anttila, L. (1997). Visualization of clinical data with neural networks, case study: Polycystic ovary syndrome. *International Journal of Medical Informatics, 44*(2), 145–155.
125. Kumar, H. P., & Srinivasan, S. (2014). Classification of ovary abnormality using the probabilistic neural network (PNN). *Technology and Health Care, 22*(6), 857–865.
126. Madhumitha, J., Kalaiyarasi, M., & Ram, S. S. (2021, May). Automated polycystic ovarian syndrome identification with follicle recognition. In *2021 3rd international conference on signal processing and communication (ICPSC)* (pp. 98–102). IEEE.

127. Ho, C. H., Chang, C. M., Li, H. Y., Shen, H. Y., Lieu, F. K., & Wang, P. S. G. (2020). Dysregulated immunological and metabolic functions discovered by a polygenic integrative analysis for PCOS. *Reproductive BioMedicine Online, 40*(1), 160–167.
128. Gopalakrishnan, C., & Iyapparaja, M. (2021). Multilevel thresholding-based follicle detection and classification of polycystic ovary syndrome from the ultrasound images using machine learning. *International Journal of System Assurance Engineering and Management*, 1–8.
129. Dong, F., Deng, D., Chen, H., Cheng, W., Li, Q., Luo, R., & Ding, S. (2015). Serum metabolomics study of polycystic ovary syndrome based on UPLC-QTOF-MS coupled with a pattern recognition approach. *Analytical and Bioanalytical Chemistry, 407*, 4683–4695.
130. Deshpande, S. S., & Wakankar, A. (2014, May). Automated detection of polycystic ovarian syndrome using follicle recognition. In *2014 IEEE international conference on advanced communications, control and computing technologies* (pp. 1341–1346). IEEE.
131. Denny, A., Raj, A., Ashok, A., Ram, C. M., & George, R. (2019, October). i-hope: Detection and prediction system for polycystic ovary syndrome (pcos) using machine learning techniques. In *TENCON 2019–2019 IEEE region 10 conference (TENCON)* (pp. 673–678). IEEE.
132. Deng, Y., Wang, Y., & Shen, Y. (2011). An automated diagnostic system of polycystic ovary syndrome based on object growing. *Artificial Intelligence in Medicine, 51*(3), 199–209.
133. Dapas, M., Lin, F. T., Nadkarni, G. N., Sisk, R., Legro, R. S., Urbanek, M., Hayes, M. G., & Dunaif, A. (2020). Distinct subtypes of polycystic ovary syndrome with novel genetic associations: An unsupervised, phenotypic clustering analysis. *PLoS Medicine, 17*(6), e1003132.
134. Che, Q., Liu, M., Xu, J., Liu, Y., Cao, X., Dong, X., & Liu, S. (2019). Characterization of circular RNA expression profiles in cumulus cells from patients with polycystic ovary syndrome. *Fertility and Sterility, 111*(6), 1243–1251.
135. Cheng, J. J., & Mahalingaiah, S. (2019). Data mining polycystic ovary morphology in electronic medical record ultrasound reports. *Fertility Research and Practice, 5*, 1–7.
136. Zhang, X., Liang, B., Zhang, J., Hao, X., Xu, X., Chang, H. M., Leung, P. C., & Tan, J. (2021). Raman spectroscopy of follicular fluid and plasma with machine-learning algorithms for polycystic ovary syndrome screening. *Molecular and Cellular Endocrinology, 523*, 111139.
137. Xie, N. N., Wang, F. F., Zhou, J., Liu, C., & Qu, F. (2020). Establishment and analysis of a combined diagnostic model of polycystic ovary syndrome with random forest and artificial neural network. *BioMed Research International, 2020*(1), 2613091.
138. Thakre, V., Vedpathak, S., Thakre, K., & Sonawani, S. (2020). PCOcare: PCOS detection and prediction using machine learning algorithms. *Bioscience Biotechnology Research Communications, 13*(14), 240–244.
139. Vikas, B., Anuhya, B. S., Bhargav, K. S., Sarangi, S., & Chilla, M. (2018). Application of the apriori algorithm for prediction of Polycystic Ovarian Syndrome (PCOS). In *Information systems design and intelligent applications: proceedings of fourth international conference INDIA 2017* (pp. 934–944). Springer Singapore.
140. Setiawati, E., Wirayuda, T. A., & Astuti, W. (2016). A classification of polycystic ovary syndrome based on ultrasound images using supervised learning and particle swarm optimization. *Advanced Science Letters, 22*(8), 1997–2001.
141. Rihana, S., Moussallem, H., Skaf, C., & Yaacoub, C. (2013, September). Automated algorithm for ovarian cysts detection in ultrasonogram. In *2013 2nd international conference on advances in biomedical engineering* (pp. 219–222). IEEE.
142. Deng, Y., Wang, Y., & Chen, P. (2008, August). Automated detection of polycystic ovary syndrome from ultrasound images. In *2008 30th annual international conference of the IEEE engineering in medicine and biology society* (pp. 4772–4775). IEEE.
143. Roy, D. G., & Alvi, P. A. (2022). Artificial intelligence in diagnosis of polycystic ovarian syndrome. In *Contemporary Issues in communication, cloud and big data analytics: Proceedings of CCB 2020* (pp. 453–463). Springer Singapore.
144. Sumathi, M., Chitra, P., Prabha, R. S., & Srilatha, K. (2021, February). Study and detection of PCOS related diseases using CNN. In *IOP conference series: Materials science and engineering* (Vol. 1070, No. 1, p. 012062). IOP Publishing.

145. Dewi, R. M., Adiwijaya, Wisesty, U. N., & Jondri. (2018, March). Classification of polycystic ovary based on ultrasound images using competitive neural network. In *Journal of Physics: Conference Series* (Vol. 971, p. 012005). IOP Publishing.
146. Hosain, A. S., Mehedi, M. H. K., & Kabir, I. E. (2022, October). Pconet: A convolutional neural network architecture to detect polycystic ovary syndrome (pcos) from ovarian ultrasound images. In *2022 International Conference on Engineering and Emerging Technologies (ICEET)* (pp. 1–6). IEEE.
147. S. Bhosale, L. Joshi, & A. Shivsharan, PCOS (Polycystic Ovarian NDROME) Detection Using Deep Learning, May 2022.
148. Alamoudi, A., Khan, I. U., Aslam, N., Alqahtani, N., Alsaif, H. S., Al Dandan, O., Al Gadeeb, M., & Al Bahrani, R. (2023). A deep learning fusion approach to diagnosis the polycystic ovary syndrome (pcos). *Applied Computational Intelligence and Soft Computing, 2023*(1), 9686697.
149. Chitra, P., Srilatha, K., Sumathi, M., Jayasudha, F. V., Bernatin, T., & Jagadeesh, M. (2023, March). Classification of ultrasound pcos image using deep learning based hybrid models. In *2023 second international conference on electronics and renewable systems (ICEARS)* (pp. 1389–1394). IEEE.
150. Krishnaveni, V., Deepa, C., Cindhu, R. S., & Santhiya, K. G. (2020). An ANN based Screener for the early diagnose of Polycystic Ovarian Syndrome in adolescent and young women. *India, March-2020.*
151. Thara, L., & Divya, T. M. (2021). Detection and prediction system for polycystic ovary syndrome using structural normalized square similarity detection approach. *NVEO-Natural Volatiles & Essential Oils Journal|NVEO*, 2834–2842.
152. Maheswari, K., Baranidharan, T., Karthik, S., & Sumathi, T. (2021). Modelling of F3I based feature selection approach for PCOS classification and prediction. *Journal of Ambient Intelligence and Humanized Computing, 12*, 1349–1362.
153. Hassan, M. M., & Mirza, T. (2020). Comparative analysis of machine learning algorithms in diagnosis of polycystic ovarian syndrome. *International Journal of Computers and Applications, 975*(8887).
154. Nandipati, S. C., & Ying, C. X. (2020). Polycystic Ovarian Syndrome (PCOS) classification and feature selection by machine learning techniques. *Applied Mathematics and Computational Intelligence (AMCI), 9*, 65–74.
155. Alagarsamy, M., Shanmugam, N., Mani, D. P., Thayumanavan, M., Sundari, K. K., & Suriyan, K. (2023). Detection of polycystic syndrome in ovary using machine learning algorithm. *International Journal of Intelligent Systems and Applications in Engineering, 11*(1), 246–253.
156. Nsugbe, E. (2023). An artificial intelligence-based decision support system for early diagnosis of polycystic ovaries syndrome. *Healthcare Analytics, 3*, Article 100164.
157. Chakraborty, S. (2022). Multi-disease detection using hybrid machine learning. *Scholars Journal of Engineering and Technology, 10*, 271–278.
158. Khanna, V. V., Chadaga, K., Sampathila, N., Prabhu, S., Bhandage, V., & Hegde, G. K. (2023). A distinctive explainable machine learning framework for detection of polycystic ovary syndrome. *Applied System Innovation, 6*(2), 32.
159. Vasavi, R. R., Prathibha, S. P., Valiveti, H., Maringanti, S., & Parsa, A. (2023, January). Polycystic ovary syndrome monitoring using machine learning. In *2023 International Conference on Intelligent Data Communication Technologies and Internet of Things (IDCIoT)* (pp. 1013–1019). IEEE.
160. Aggarwal, S., & Pandey, K. (2023). Early identification of PCOS with commonly known diseases: Obesity, diabetes, high blood pressure and heart disease using machine learning techniques. *Expert Systems with Applications, 217*, Article 119532.
161. Hdaib, D., Almajali, N., Alquran, H., Mustafa, W. A., Al-Azzawi, W., & Alkhayyat, A. (2022, May). Detection of polycystic ovary syndrome (PCOS) using machine learning algorithms. In *2022 5th international conference on engineering technology and its applications (IICETA)* (pp. 532–536). IEEE.

162. Danaei Mehr, H., & Polat, H. (2022). Diagnosis of polycystic ovary syndrome through different machine learning and feature selection techniques. *Health and Technology, 12*(1), 137–150.
163. Bhat, S. A., & Gupta, R., National College of Ireland Project Submission Sheet School of Computing, May 2021.
164. Inan, M. S. K., Ulfath, R. E., Alam, F. I., Bappee, F. K., & Hasan, R. (2021, January). Improved sampling and feature selection to support extreme gradient boosting for PCOS diagnosis. In *2021 IEEE 11th annual computing and communication workshop and conference (CCWC)* (pp. 1046–1050). IEEE.
165. Alshakrani, S., Hilal, S., & Zeki, A. M. (2022, October). Hybrid machine learning algorithms for polycystic ovary syndrome detection. In *2022 international conference on data analytics for business and industry (ICDABI)* (pp. 160–164). IEEE.
166. Rahman, M. M., Islam, A., Islam, F., Zaman, M., Islam, M. R., Sakib, M. S. A., & Babu, H. M. H. (2024). Empowering early detection: A web-based machine learning approach for PCOS prediction. *Informatics in Medicine Unlocked, 47*, Article 101500.
167. Suha, S. A., & Islam, M. N. (2022). An extended machine learning technique for polycystic ovary syndrome detection using ovary ultrasound image. *Scientific Reports, 12*(1), 17123.
168. Adla, Y. A. A., Raydan, D. G., Charaf, M. Z. J., Saad, R. A., Nasreddine, J., & Diab, M. O. (2021, October). Automated detection of polycystic ovary syndrome using machine learning techniques. In *2021 Sixth international conference on advances in biomedical engineering (ICABME)* (pp. 208–212). IEEE.
169. Zigarelli, A., Jia, Z., & Lee, H. (2022). Machine-aided self-diagnostic prediction models for polycystic ovary syndrome: Observational study. *JMIR Formative Research, 6*(3), Article e29967.
170. Chattot, C., Huchon, C., Paternostre, A., Du Cheyron, J., Chouillard, E., & Fauconnier, A. (2019). ENDORECT: A preoperative score to accurately predict rectosigmoid involvement in patients with endometriosis. *Human Reproduction Open, 2019*(2), hoz007.
171. Guo, Z., Feng, P., Chen, X., Tang, R., & Yu, Q. (2020). Developing preoperative nomograms to predict any-stage and stage III-IV endometriosis in infertile women. *Frontiers in Medicine, 7*, Article 570483.
172. Nnoaham, K. E., Hummelshoj, L., Kennedy, S. H., Jenkinson, C., Zondervan, K. T., & World Endometriosis Research Foundation Women's Health Symptom Survey Consortium. (2012). Developing symptom-based predictive models of endometriosis as a clinical screening tool: results from a multicenter study. *Fertility and Sterility, 98*(3), 692–701.
173. Li, B., Wang, S., Duan, H., Wang, Y., & Guo, Z. (2021). Discovery of gene module acting on ubiquitin-mediated proteolysis pathway by co-expression network analysis for endometriosis. *Reproductive BioMedicine Online, 42*(2), 429–441.
174. Akter, S., Xu, D., Nagel, S. C., Bromfield, J. J., Pelch, K. E., Wilshire, G. B., & Joshi, T. (2020). GenomeForest: An ensemble machine learning classifier for endometriosis. *AMIA Summits on Translational Science Proceedings, 2020*, 33.
175. Perrotta, A. R., Borrelli, G. M., Martins, C. O., Kallas, E. G., Sanabani, S. S., Griffith, L. G., Alm, E. J., & Abrao, M. S. (2020). The vaginal microbiome as a tool to predict rASRM stage of disease in endometriosis: a pilot study. *Reproductive Sciences, 27*, 1064–1073.
176. Akter, S., Xu, D., Nagel, S. C., Bromfield, J. J., Pelch, K., Wilshire, G. B., & Joshi, T. (2019). Machine learning classifiers for endometriosis using transcriptomics and methylomics data. *Frontiers in Genetics, 10*, 766.
177. Tamaresis, J. S., Irwin, J. C., Goldfien, G. A., Rabban, J. T., Burney, R. O., Nezhat, C., DePaolo, L. V., & Giudice, L. C. (2014). Molecular classification of endometriosis and disease stage using high-dimensional genomic data. *Endocrinology, 155*(12), 4986-4999.
178. Bendifallah, S., Puchar, A., Suisse, S., Delbos, L., Poilblanc, M., Descamps, P., Golfier, F., Touboul, C., Dabi, Y., & Daraï, E. (2022). Machine learning algorithms as new screening approach for patients with endometriosis. *Scientific Reports, 12*(1), 639.
179. Vesale, E., Roman, H., Abo, C., Benoit, L., Tuech, J. J., Darai, E., & Bendifallah, S. (2021). Predictive approach in managing voiding dysfunction after surgery for deep endometriosis: A personalized nomogram. *International Urogynecology Journal, 32*, 1205–1212.

180. Benoit, L., Boujenah, J., Poncelet, C., Grynberg, M., Carbillon, L., Timoh, K. N., Touleimat, S., D'argent, E.M., Jayot, A., Owen, C., Lavoue, V., & Bendifallah, S. (2019). Predicting the likelihood of a live birth for women with endometriosis-related infertility. *European Journal of Obstetrics & Gynecology and Reproductive Biology, 242*, 56–62.
181. Lafay Pillet, M. C., Huchon, C., Santulli, P., Borghese, B., Chapron, C., & Fauconnier, A. (2014). A clinical score can predict associated deep infiltrating endometriosis before surgery for an endometrioma. *Human Reproduction, 29*(8), 1666–1676.
182. Ballester, M., Oppenheimer, A., Mathieu d'Argent, E., Touboul, C., Antoine, J. M., Coutant, C., & Daraï, E. (2012). Nomogram to predict pregnancy rate after ICSI–IVF cycle in patients with endometriosis. *Human Reproduction, 27*(2), 451–456.
183. Chapron, C., Barakat, H., Fritel, X., Dubuisson, J. B., Bréart, G., & Fauconnier, A. (2005). Presurgical diagnosis of posterior deep infiltrating endometriosis based on a standardized questionnaire. *Human Reproduction, 20*(2), 507–513.
184. Wang, Y. F., Chang, M. Y., Chiang, R. D., Hwang, L. J., Lee, C. M., & Wang, Y. H. (2013). Mining medical data: A case study of endometriosis. *Journal of Medical Systems, 37*, 1–7.
185. Parlatan, U., Inanc, M. T., Ozgor, B. Y., Oral, E., Bastu, E., Unlu, M. B., & Basar, G. (2019). Raman spectroscopy as a non-invasive diagnostic technique for endometriosis. *Scientific Reports, 9*(1), 19795.
186. Braga, D. P., Montani, D. A., Setti, A. S., Turco, E. G. L., Oliveira-Silva, D., & Borges, E., Jr. (2019). Metabolomic profile as a noninvasive adjunct tool for the diagnosis of Grades III and IV endometriosis-related infertility. *Molecular Reproduction and Development, 86*(8), 1044–1052.
187. Dutta, M., Joshi, M., Srivastava, S., Lodh, I., Chakravarty, B., & Chaudhury, K. (2012). A metabonomics approach as a means for identification of potential biomarkers for early diagnosis of endometriosis. *Molecular BioSystems, 8*(12), 3281–3287.
188. Ghazi, N., Arjmand, M., Akbari, Z., Mellati, A. O., Saheb-Kashaf, H., & Zamani, Z. (2016). 1H NMR-based metabolomics approaches as non-invasive tools for diagnosis of endometriosis. *International Journal of Reproductive Biomedicine, 14*(1), 1.
189. Wang, L., Liu, H. Y., Shi, H. H., Lang, J. H., & Sun, W. (2014). Urine peptide patterns for non-invasive diagnosis of endometriosis: A preliminary prospective study. *European Journal of Obstetrics & Gynecology and Reproductive Biology, 177*, 23–28.
190. Wölfler, M. M., Schwamborn, K., Otten, D., Hornung, D., Liu, H., & Rath, W. (2009). Mass spectrometry and serum pattern profiling for analyzing the individual risk for endometriosis: Promising insights? *Fertility and Sterility, 91*(6), 2331–2337.
191. Fassbender, A., Waelkens, E., Verbeeck, N., Kyama, C. M., Bokor, A., Vodolazkaia, A., Van de Plas, R., Meuleman, C., Peeraer, K., Tomassetti, C., Gevaert, O., & D'Hooghe, T. (2012). Proteomics analysis of plasma for early diagnosis of endometriosis. *Obstetrics & Gynecology, 119*(2 Part 1), 276–285.
192. Fassbender, A., Verbeeck, N., Börnigen, D., Kyama, C. M., Bokor, A., Vodolazkaia, A., Peeraer, K., Tomassetti, C., Meuleman, C., Gevaert, O., Van de Plas, R., & D'Hooghe, T. M. (2012). Combined mRNA microarray and proteomic analysis of eutopic endometrium of women with and without endometriosis. *Human Reproduction, 27*(7), 2020–2029.
193. Wang, L., Zheng, W., Ding, X. Y., Yu, J. K., Jiang, W. Z., & Zhang, S. Z. (2010). Identification biomarkers of eutopic endometrium in endometriosis using artificial neural networks and protein fingerprinting. *Fertility and Sterility, 93*(7), 2460–2462.
194. Wang, L., Zheng, W., Mu, L., & Zhang, S. Z. (2008). Identifying biomarkers of endometriosis using serum protein fingerprinting and artificial neural networks. *International Journal of Gynecology & Obstetrics, 101*(3), 253–258.
195. Maicas, G., Leonardi, M., Avery, J., Panuccio, C., Carneiro, G., Hull, M. L., & Condous, G. (2021). Deep learning to diagnose pouch of Douglas obliteration with ultrasound sliding sign. *Reproduction and Fertility, 2*(4), 236–243.
196. Guerriero, S., Pascual, M., Ajossa, S., Neri, M., Musa, E., Graupera, B., et al. (2021). Artificial intelligence (AI) in the detection of rectosigmoid deep endometriosis. *European Journal of Obstetrics & Gynecology and Reproductive Biology, 261*, 29–33.

197. Reid, S., Lu, C., & Condous, G. (2015). Can we improve the prediction of pouch of Douglas obliteration in women with suspected endometriosis using ultrasound-based models? A multicenter prospective observational study. *Acta Obstetricia et Gynecologica Scandinavica, 94*(12), 1297–1306.
198. Shahzad, A., Mushtaq, A., Sabeeh, A. Q., Ghadi, Y. Y., Mushtaq, Z., Arif, S., Ur Rehman, M.Z., Qureshi, M.F., & Jamil, F. (2023, May). Automated uterine fibroids detection in ultrasound images using deep convolutional neural networks. In *Healthcare* (Vol. 11, No. 10, p. 1493). MDPI.
199. Zhang, J., Yang, C., Gong, C., Zhou, Y., Li, C., & Li, F. (2022). Magnetic resonance imaging parameter-based machine learning for prognosis prediction of high-intensity focused ultrasound ablation of uterine fibroids. *International Journal of Hyperthermia, 39*(1), 835–846.
200. Luo, Y. H., Xi, I. L., Wang, R., Abdallah, H. O., Wu, J., Vance, A. Z., Chang, K., Kohi, M., Jones, L., Reddy, S. and Zhang, Z.S., & Shlansky-Goldberg, R. (2020). Deep learning based on MR imaging for predicting outcome of uterine fibroid embolization. *Journal of Vascular and Interventional Radiology, 31*(6), 1010–1017.
201. Girija, D. K., & Varshney, M. (2022). Proposed model to detect uterine fibroid by using data mining techniques. *Journal of Positive School Psychology, 6*(2), 2062–2065.
202. Huo, T., Li, L., Chen, X., Wang, Z., Zhang, X., Liu, S., Huang, J., Zhang, J., Yang, Q., Wu, W., Xie, Y., & Deng, K. (2023). Artificial intelligence-aided method to detect uterine fibroids in ultrasound images: A retrospective study. *Scientific Reports, 13*(1), 3714.
203. Dilna, K. T., Anitha, J., Angelopoulou, A., Kapetanios, E., Chaussalet, T., & Hemanth, D. J. (2022, June). Classification of uterine fibroids in ultrasound images using deep learning model. In *International Conference on Computational Science* (pp. 50–56). Springer International Publishing.
204. Yang, T., Yuan, L., Li, P., & Liu, P. (2023). Real-time automatic assisted detection of uterine fibroid in ultrasound images using a deep learning detector. *Ultrasound in Medicine & Biology, 49*(7), 1616–1626.
205. Suomi, V., Komar, G., Sainio, T., Joronen, K., Perheentupa, A., & Blanco Sequeiros, R. (2019). Comprehensive feature selection for classifying the treatment outcome of high-intensity ultrasound therapy in uterine fibroids. *Scientific Reports, 9*(1), 10907.
206. Sumathy, V., Rexline, S. J., & Gowri, T. D. (2022). Decision support tool for uterine fibroids treatment with machine learning algorithms—A study. *International Journal of Scientific Research Publication, 12*, 442–449.
207. Tang, C. M., Liu, D., & Yu, X. (2020). MRI image segmentation system of uterine fibroids based on AR-Unet network. *American Scientific Research Journal for Engineering, Technology, and Sciences, 71*, 1–10.
208. Sadullaeva, S. A., Sadullaeva, U. A., Artikova, M. A., Aripovaz, D., & Radjabova, M. R. (2022). Analysis of detection and segmentation of uterine fibroids between uzbek women. *NeuroQuantology, 20*(10), 83.
209. Theis, M., Tonguc, T., Savchenko, O., Nowak, S., Block, W., Recker, F., Essler, M., Mustea, A., Attenberger, U., Marinova, M., & Sprinkart, A. M. (2023). Deep learning enables automated MRI-based estimation of uterine volume also in patients with uterine fibroids undergoing high-intensity focused ultrasound therapy. *Insights into Imaging, 14*(1), 1.
210. Luo, X., et al. Segmentation and registration of ultrasound images of uterine fibroids for usghifu. In *2021 14th international congress on image and signal processing, biomedical engineering and informatics (CISP-BMEI)*. IEEE, 2021.
211. Yang, C., Huang, Q., Ji, X., & Bai, J. (2020, July). Fusion of multiple-angles intraoperative us images and pretreatment mr images for usghifu treatment of uterine fibroid: Retrospective evaluation based on clinical dataset. In *2020 42nd annual international conference of the IEEE engineering in medicine & biology society (EMBC)* (pp. 5236–5239). IEEE.
212. Kurata, Y., Nishio, M., Kido, A., Fujimoto, K., Yakami, M., Isoda, H., & Togashi, K. (2019). Automatic segmentation of the uterus on MRI using a convolutional neural network. *Computers in Biology and Medicine, 114*, Article 103438.

213. Rundo, L., Tangherloni, A., Cazzaniga, P., Nobile, M. S., Russo, G., Gilardi, M. C., et al. (2019). A novel framework for MR image segmentation and quantification by using MedGA. *Computer Methods and Programs in Biomedicine, 176*, 159–172.
214. Rundo, L., Militello, C., Vitabile, S., Casarino, C., Russo, G., Midiri, M., & Gilardi, M. C. (2016). Combining split-and-merge and multi-seed region growing algorithms for uterine fibroid segmentation in MRgFUS treatments. *Medical & Biological Engineering & Computing, 54*, 1071–1084.
215. Prabakar, S., Porkumaran, K., & Guna Sundari, J. (2014). Uterine fibroid segmentation and measurement based on morphological functions in graphical vision assistant tool. In *Emerging research in electronics, computer science and technology: Proceedings of international conference, ICERECT 2012* (pp. 357–366). Springer India.
216. Ning, G., Zhang, X., Zhang, Q., Wang, Z., & Liao, H. (2020). Real-time and multimodality image-guided intelligent HIFU therapy for uterine fibroid. *Theranostics, 10*(10), 4676.
217. Sundar, S., & Sumathy, S. (2022). Transfer learning approach in deep neural networks for uterine fibroid detection. *International Journal of Computational Science and Engineering, 25*(1), 52–63.
218. Zhao, A., Du, X., Wang, S., Wang, W., Yuan, S., Ma, W., Yan, W., Shen, W., & Zhu, X. (2022, October). A CNN-transformer hybrid network for recognizing uterine fibroids. In *2022 IEEE international conference on consumer electronics-Asia (ICCE-Asia)* (pp. 1–4). IEEE.
219. Zhang, Y., Wang, Z., Zhang, J., Wang, C., Wang, Y., Chen, H., Shan, L., Huo, J, Gu, J., & Ma, X. (2021). Deep learning model for classifying endometrial lesions. *Journal of Translational Medicine, 19*, 1–13.
220. Sriraam, N., Nithyashri, D., Vinodashri, L., & Niranjan, P. M. (2010, November). Detection of uterine fibroids using wavelet packet features with BPNN classifier. In *2010 IEEE EMBS conference on biomedical engineering and sciences (IECBES)* (pp. 406–409). IEEE.
221. Yang, T., Li, P., & Liu, P. (2022, December). Efficient automatic detection of uterine fibroids based on the scalable EfficientDet. In *2022 IEEE 16th international conference on anti-counterfeiting, security, and identification (ASID)* (pp. 157–160). IEEE.
222. Behboodi, B., Rivaz, H., Lalondrelle, S., & Harris, E. (2021, September). Automatic 3D ultrasound segmentation of uterus using deep learning. In *2021 IEEE international ultrasonics symposium (IUS)* (pp. 1–4). IEEE.
223. Ademola, B. J., Adebayo, I. P., & Thomas, B. O. A predictive model for the risk of infertility in women using supervised machine learning algorithms (a comparative analysis).
224. Simi, M. S., Nayaki, K. S., Parameswaran, M., & Sivadasan, S. (2017, October). Exploring female infertility using predictive analytic. In *2017 IEEE global humanitarian technology conference (GHTC)* (pp. 1–6). IEEE.
225. Aror, A., & Chouksey, P. (2017). A novel approach for women's infertility detection using data mining techniques. *International Journal of Electronics Communication and Computer Engineering, 8*, 129–133.

Chapter 5
XAI: Focusing on Fertility Assessment

5.1 Introduction

In the era of transformative tech, Explainable Artificial Intelligence (XAI) has emerged as a crucial field within AI, essential for building trust, ensuring compliance, and improving the effectiveness and reliability of intelligent systems. Over the last few years, the integration of AI into healthcare has significantly reshaped the medical landscape. Despite the well-documented advancements in AI, the incorporation of AI systems into operational applications remains uncertain due to concerns about trustworthiness [1]. To overcome these challenges, a mechanism called XAI has been developed to enhance the understandability of AI applications, making them accessible not only to domain experts but also to laypersons unfamiliar with AI's complexities [2].

Although the value of AI explainability can be analyzed from multiple perspectives, it primarily revolves around interpretability and explainability. Each process offers distinct insights into understanding AI systems. Interpretability pertains to the development of human-understandable rules that govern a system's decision-making, whereas explainability focuses on designing interfaces that enhance the accessibility and comprehensibility of AI-driven decisions [3]. XAI has the potential to elucidate the internal mechanisms of AI decision-making processes. Moreover, its applications span a wide range of AI domains, with healthcare emerging as a particularly impactful area [4].

Healthcare and medicine encompass diverse fields, including the diagnosis, prevention, and treatment of diseases. Certain areas pose significant challenges for clinicians, such as the manual analysis of X-rays, MRI, CT scans, and ultrasounds. Diagnosis extends beyond image data, as text data also plays an essential role [5]. For example, various studies have leveraged clinical and lifestyle factors to diagnose conditions like PCOS, sperm quality issues, and other fertility-related

KC. Santosh and D. G. Roy, *Artificial Intelligence for Human Fertility: Trends, Insights, and Predictions*, Studies in Computational Intelligence 1230,
https://doi.org/10.1007/978-981-95-1248-5_5

concerns. Similarly, textual data is instrumental in detecting mental health conditions, including depression, anxiety, and more. In healthcare, prevention and treatment are core components that can be both labour-intensive and time-consuming for clinicians. Effective prevention relies on early diagnosis, while successful treatment depends on accurate diagnosis. Trustworthy and transparent AI systems can significantly enhance both processes, enabling timely and precise medical interventions while reducing the burden on healthcare professionals.

Two primary types of AI applications, namely ML and DL, are predominantly implemented in healthcare. ML models are designed to carry out specific tasks by identifying clear patterns and relationships within data. Similarly, DL models, a segment of ML, are structured with multiple hidden layers, along with an input and output layer. These models require extensive datasets and high-performance computational resources to function effectively. The research community has increasingly dedicated attention to DL due to its multifunctionality, exceptional performance, strong generalization capability, and diverse applications. This has led to significant improvements over earlier ML-based models, particularly in biomedical image classification and segmentation [6].

Despite that, the distinct data requirements and capabilities of ML and DL pose challenges when handling the unique characteristics of medical data, which are diverse in nature and often limited in quantity. Both DL and ML models often operate as opaque systems, offering minimal to no transparency into the reasoning behind their predictions. As a result, clinicians struggle to understand the reasoning behind these predictions, making it difficult to verify results [7]. The opacity of AI systems has hindered widespread adoption among clinicians, who depend on evidence-based diagnoses to inform their treatment decisions. Additionally, clinicians must ensure that AI models are properly trained and that their outputs are grounded in reliable medical knowledge. Advanced AI models, such as deep neural networks, are typically trained on high-dimensional data and capture critical features. Therefore, providing clear explanations and interpretations of model outputs is crucial for improving the usability of these systems and facilitating their wider adoption in healthcare [8].

XAI refers to a set of techniques that provide insights into how an AI model generates its predictions. In essence, XAI enables users to comprehend the model's decision-making process and the reasoning behind its outputs. In the context of medical image classification, XAI can clarify how the model operates and identifies the specific image regions that most influence its predictions. By highlighting the most distinguishing features, input data can be refined using various preprocessing techniques to emphasize the attributes utilized in decision-making. The key aspects of XAI include causality, which refers to the model's ability to identify meaningful relationships between different features, and transferability, which allows the knowledge derived from XAI to be applied across different problem domains. Effective visualization of explainability is also essential, particularly when AI models serve as decision support tools in clinical practice [9]. By integrating XAI techniques into ML and DL models, AI applications in the clinical field will become more transparent, reliable, and widely accepted. Furthermore, these enhancements can contribute to continuous improvements in model performance and overall trust in AI-driven healthcare solutions [10].

AI explainability solutions designed to interpret ML models, particularly those based on post-hoc analysis, can be categorized into model-agnostic and model-specific methods. Model-agnostic approaches are versatile techniques that can be applied to virtually any ML model, regardless of its structure or training methodology. One widely used model-agnostic technique is Sensitivity Analysis (SA), which evaluates the influence of input variables on output predictions by systematically modifying input values and assessing the resulting changes in the model's output. These methods determine the sensitivity of predictions to individual input features by leveraging statistical measures such as variance, derivatives, and density. Sensitivity analysis can be performed at both a local and global level [11]. Local Sensitivity Analysis (SA) examines how small, incremental changes in input values impact the model's predictions, focusing on localized perturbations to assess the model's responsiveness. In contrast, Global Sensitivity Analysis takes a more comprehensive approach by varying input parameters across their entire range, providing a broader perspective on how different input scenarios influence the overall output. This distinction between local and global sensitivity analysis is essential for understanding the varying degrees of impact that input features have on the model's decision-making process [12].

Unlike model-agnostic approaches, model-specific methods are designed for specific ML models and cannot be applied to others. For instance, several techniques have been developed to explain deep neural networks, collectively referred to as deep network understanding and visualization. Notable methods in this category include Activation Maximization, DeConvNet, Inversion, DeepDream, Feature Visualization, and DeepLift. These techniques aim to understand how individual neurons in Convolutional Neural Networks contribute to final predictions through optimization and backpropagation [13]. Additionally, there are specialized approaches designed for explaining Graph Neural Networks and Recurrent Neural Networks. Many researchers argue that a complete understanding of a model requires insight into the reasoning behind its decisions. In this context, counterfactual reasoning has emerged as a valuable method for identifying the features that influence specific outcomes. Recent advancements have focused on hybrid approaches that enhance the transparency of AI models while retaining the power and complexity of deep learning architectures. Examples of such models include Contextual Explanation Networks, Self-Explaining Neural Networks, BagNet, and TabNet [11]. As the demand for interpretability grows among end-users, further research in this area is essential. Transparency in AI models is particularly critical in high-stakes fields such as healthcare, where the implications of AI-driven decisions can be significant.

Designing XAI models is essential for ensuring the adoption and accountability of AI systems in clinical practice. The concept of XAI can be categorized into three main approaches, as depicted in Fig. 5.1. The first is pre-modelling explainability, which uses data processing techniques to analyze and understand the datasets used for training ML models. The second approach focuses on interpretable models that are inherently transparent, enabling users to comprehend their structure and

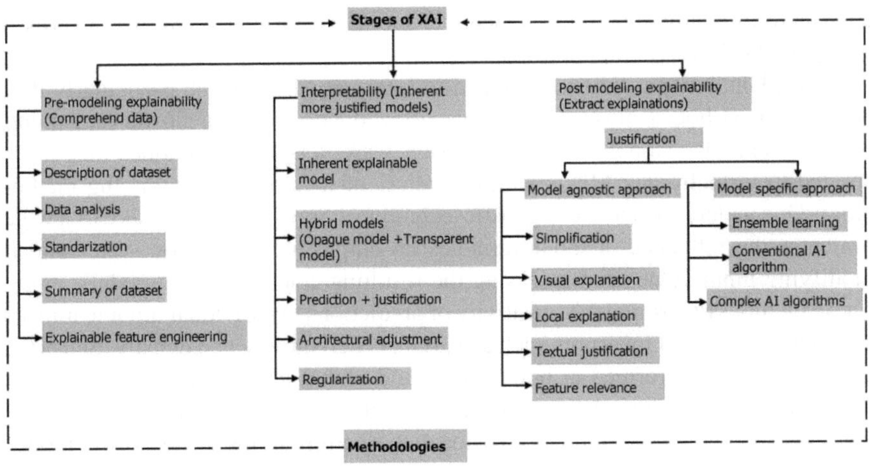

Fig. 5.1 Chart illustrating the stages of explainable AI (XAI). It is composed of three main sections: pre-modelling explainability, interpretability, and post-modelling explainability. Pre-modelling includes steps like description of dataset, data analysis, standardization, and explainable feature engineering. Interpretability involves inherent explainable models, hybrid models, prediction with justification, architectural adjustment, and regularization. Post-modelling focuses on justification through model-agnostic and model-specific approaches, including simplification, visual explanation, local explanation, textual justification, feature relevance, ensemble learning, and complex AI algorithms. The chart is framed within a dashed border labelled "Methodologies"

behaviour. The third is post-modelling explainability, which enhances the clarity of black-box ML models through techniques such as visualization, textual explanations, simplification, and feature relevance analysis.

As per European Union has outlined seven key requirements for XAI models, including human oversight, technical robustness, privacy, transparency, fairness, social well-being, and accountability [14]. These requirements focus on ensuring the security of AI systems in healthcare, addressing risks like network attacks and biases. Integrity and accountability are crucial, as ethical concerns about AI's impact on healthcare professionals and patients continue to emerge. Efforts to mitigate biases, especially in recognition tasks, are necessary to ensure fairness and avoid inconsistent outcomes in clinical settings. Explainability plays a vital role in maintaining responsibility and addressing these challenges [15].

5.2 Methods

The methods of XAI can be classified into six primary categories: feature-oriented schemes, global schemes, concept systems, surrogate systems, local pixel-based schemes, and human-centric schemes.

Feature-Oriented Schemes:

Feature-oriented techniques work on the Shapley Additive Explanation (SHAP) strategy, which is developed based on game theory. This game theory estimates the contribution of each participant in a cooperative game and uses the Shapley value to represent the contribution of each participant [16]. Consequently, the rewards of the game are distributed according to the Shapley value. Using this concept ML model outcomes can be explained, where the inputs of a black-box model (AI model) are considered contributors to the model's output, and the Shapley value of each variable represents its contribution to the output. This process can be used to justify the model's output and is regarded as interpreting a black-box model.

SHAP is a widely used approach, though its estimation is complex from both theoretical and computational perspectives. For a given example, $x = [x_1, \ldots, x_n]$, the impact of each feature x_j to the prediction $f(x)$ of a ML system is calculated using Shapley values. This is done by considering $\{x_1, \ldots, x_n\}$ as contributors in a coalition game, represented as $(v, N = \{x_1, .., x_n\}$. The payoff function v: $2^N \rightarrow R$, $v(\emptyset) = 0$ maps subsets of attributes (cooperative players) to real numbers. For a segment of attributes S, $v(S)$ represents the expected total of payoffs resulting from the cooperation of attributes in S. Once the payoff function is established, the Shapley value of the j-th feature ($\emptyset_j$ (v)) is computed as the mean marginal impact of the j-th attribute to the payoff, as expressed below:

$$\emptyset_j(v) = \sum_{S \subseteq N\{j\}} w_{s,N}(v(S \cup \{j\} - v(S)). \tag{5.1}$$

The summation is carried out over all feasible coalitions S in which the j-th player is eliminated. Additionally, $w_{s,N}$ serves as the weight component, which is calculated as

$$w_{s,N} = \frac{|S|!(|N| - |S| - 1)!}{|N|!}, \tag{5.2}$$

where $|S|$ denotes the cardinality of the segment S, and $w_{s,N}$, N is the inverse of the multinomial coefficient, expressing the number of distinct paths to form a coalition via segment S of N while removing the j-th feature. Using the Shapley values $\{\emptyset_j(v), j = 1, \ldots, n\}$, the SHAP explanation can be derived as shown in Eq. (5.3):

$$g(z') = \emptyset_0 + \sum_{j=1}^{n} \emptyset_j z_{j'}, \tag{5.3}$$

where $z' = [z_{1'}, .., z_{n'}] \in \{0, 1\}^n$ is a vector of binary values, where $z_{j'} = 0$, indicates that the j-th feature is omitted from the coalition, and $z_{j'} = 1$ signifies that the j-th feature is included in the coalition. Additionally, $\emptyset_0 = E[f(x)]$ represents the average predicted value calculated across all attributes.

Optimizing the implementatioof the SHAP method for specific model types remains challenging, despite its applicability across various models. Convolutional

Neural Networks (CNNs) often employ Class Activation Maps (CAMs), which represent a weighted linear combination of distinct spatial patterns associated with each class in an image. Prior to the output layer, the final convolutional attribute map is subjected to global average pooling, generating input attributes for a fully connected layer and outputs for the loss function. By backprojecting the output weights onto the preceding convolutional layer, CAMs generate a heatmap of the input image, highlighting regions that significantly influence the CNN's decision-making process. However, CAMs cannot be applied to fully Convolutional Neural Networks or pretrained models that deviate from specific architectural requirements. CAM and Grad-CAM are based on the premise that, for a given class c [17], the network's final score f^c can be represented as outlined in Eq. (5.4):

$$Y^c = \sum_k w_k^c \sum_i \sum_j A_{ij}^K. \tag{5.4}$$

In this context, Y^c denotes the final score, w_k^c represents the weight associated with A^k which is the k-th attribute map of the final convolutional layer, and A_{ij}^K refers to the value at row I and column j of A^k. Using Eq. (5.1), the saliency map value for class ccc at each location (i, j) is computed as specified in Eq. (5.5). The value L_{ij}^c represents the significance of location (i, j) for class c, with L^c providing a visual explanation for the class c predicted by the network. In the CAM approach, weight values w_k^c are obtained by training individual linear classifiers for each class:

$$L_{ij}^c = \sum_k w_k^c A_{ij}^k. \tag{5.5}$$

However, CAM assumes that the penultimate layer of the CNN utilizes global average pooling, which is not always applicable. Grad-CAM was introduced to address these limitations, showing that the weight values w_k^c for each feature A^k can be calculated as outlined in Eq. (5.6):

$$w_k^c = \frac{1}{z} \sum_i \sum_j \frac{\partial Y^c}{\partial A_{ij}^k}, \tag{5.6}$$

where z represents the number of pixels in A^k. Despite addressing some of the issues of the CAM method, Grad-CAM still has limitations, such as its inability to accurately localize objects when the input image contains multiple instances with the same class label. Additionally, the unweighted averaging in Eq. (5.2) results in the localization of only parts of objects, rather than their full extent. To address these drawbacks, Grad-CAM++ was introduced, where the global averaging in Eq. (5.2) is reformulated as shown in Eq. (5.7):

$$w_k^c = \sum_i \sum_j \alpha_{ij}^{kc} \text{relu}\left(\frac{\partial Y^c}{\partial A_{ij}^k}\right), \quad (5.7)$$

where α_{ij}^{kc} is the weight associated with the pixel (i, j) in the k-th feature map A^k. By using Eq. (5.6), w_k^c effectively captures the significance of the feature map Ak through a weighted average of partial derivatives, unlike Eq. (5.5), which employs unweighted averaging.

These applications are used in the post-modelling phase of XAI, where they effectively link decision-making to specific features and explain the "how" and "why" behind the model's conclusions. This is especially crucial in healthcare, where understanding the reasoning behind an AI's decision is as important as the decision itself.

Global schemes:

Global Attribution Mappings (GAMs) in XAI are powerful techniques that provide in-depth insights into the decision-making processes of machine learning models, particularly neural networks. GAMs help to uncover the global relationships between features across a broad range of inputs, offering a clearer understanding of how various input features collectively influence a model's behaviour. These mappings generate a pairwise rank distance matrix to capture complex interactions among attributes and apply K-medoids clustering to group similar local features, enhancing mapping accuracy. Each cluster is illustrated by a "medoid," which serves as a point of reference for constructing a global attribution by synthesizing the patterns within the cluster. This process allows GAMs to explore the unique characteristics of different sample groups, improving the interpretability of neural networks. For the most frequently predicted class by the model, GAMs create a standardized heatmap using a gradient-based saliency map, highlighting pixels with high activation levels that significantly influence the model's decision-making [18]. While gradient-based saliency maps are limited to providing insights into model diagnostics, deep attribute maps are used to improve the explainability of these algorithms. The system's prediction is visualized as a heatmap, where the significant features of the output gradient are multiplied by relevant input data, enabling comparisons with other saliency-based explanation models and enhancing transparency in understanding the model's reasoning [19].

Concept systems:

Concept Models in XAI are techniques designed to enhance the interpretability and transparency of machine learning models by linking their internal states to human-understandable concepts. These models bridge the gap between complex systems, such as deep neural networks, and human decision-making by making model behaviour more accessible. A notable example is Concept Activation Vectors (CAVs), which represent the internal state of a neural network in a human-readable format. CAVs are calculated using directional derivatives to assess the sensitivity of a system's output to specific concepts, capturing how predictions change when a concept varies. Alternatively, CAVs can be computed by determining a hyperplane that separates activation values of a specific concept from random examples, with the normal vector of this hyperplane representing the CAV [20]. The vector's direction indicates how the network aligns with the concept, offering insights into its interpretation. Widely used in healthcare, CAVs support tasks like image classification, disease forecasting, and diagnostics, including diabetic retinopathy, tumour detection, pulmonary disease analysis, cardiovascular risk assessment, and cancer detection, making machine learning systems more transparent and trustworthy in critical applications.

Surrogate systems:

The surrogate model is a simplified, interpretable version of the black-box model, designed to replicate its behaviour within the local region around a specific input instance. In the Local Interpretable Model-Agnostic Explanation (LIME) approach, the surrogate model plays a key role in providing explanations for the predictions made by complex black-box machine learning models. LIME generates locally optimal explanations by using an interpretable surrogate model to approximate the black-box classifier's behaviour. While describing the intricate workings of black-box models can be difficult, LIME makes it possible to understand their behaviour for selective input samples. The approach begins by altering parts of an input sample to create a set of perturbed instances that are similar, but not identical, to the original input. The nature of these perturbations depends on the input type. Through this approach, LIME allows users to create an interpretable model that approximates the classifier's behaviour around the selected data sample [21]. The most widespread application of LIME is in disease determination, such as fertility, Alzheimer's, diabetes, etc.

Local, pixel-based schemes:

Local pixel-based methods analyze how individual pixels or small regions of an image contribute to the predictions of machine learning models, such as deep neural networks, by generating interpretable explanations that highlight the most influential input features. LRP is a popular technique in this domain, working by backpropagating the system's output across its layers to compute the relevance of each input feature, producing heatmaps that display the contribution of specific pixels to the model's decision [22]. LRP is particularly valuable in medical applications, such as explaining neural network-based diagnoses of many diseases using structural MRI data, and in visualizing pixel-level contributions in kernel-based classifiers applied to Bag of Words models. However, challenges arise in computing gradients locally, particularly in identifying suitable reference points, underscoring the need for methods to define reference points within a predetermined neighbourhood for more accurate gradient calculations.

Human-Centric schemes:

The application of AI is widespread across domains such as healthcare, finance, law, and autonomous vehicles. It is crucial for these systems to have decision-making processes that are understandable and trustworthy to users. To address this need, a new approach known as human-centric methods has recently been proposed. The primary goal of this XAI approach is to serve humans effectively, responsibly, and transparently. Numerous articles have been published highlighting the shift from traditional AI to XAI, demonstrating the societal benefits of this transition. Furthermore, humans often rely on similarity to relate new data to previously learned and aggregated prototypes, whereas statistical methods typically use averages as their foundation [23].

5.3 XAI Tools

Plenty of literature has found that it is correlated with XAI in healthcare applications. This research focused on different aspects of the XAI topic. Many open-source platforms have been utilized by the researchers to support different modelling states which we discussed in the earlier section. Leading companies such as Google, Microsoft, and Oracle have increasingly focused on incorporating XAI into their ecosystems, underscoring its rising significance in the current environment.

The seven most widely used tools for analyzing the behaviour of AI models include AI Fairness 360, What-If Tool, Skater, H2O platform, Model Interpretability, Distill, and ELI5. These tools are primarily used during the post-modelling stage of XAI. Table 5.1 presents a quick overview of XAI tools.

AI fairness 360:

AI Fairness 360 (AIF360), an open-access library designed by IBM in 2019, is designed to detect and mitigate bias in ML models and datasets. Available in both Python and R, AIF360 offers an extensive collection of tools for identifying fairness concerns and applying mitigation techniques throughout the ML lifecycle. Its flexibility allows users to address bias in datasets during the pre-modelling stage and in trained models during the post-modelling stage. Widely adopted across various domains, AIF360 has proven to be a valuable resource for fostering ethical AI practices. By facilitating thorough fairness assessments and interventions, it enhances the transparency, accountability, and inclusivity of ML systems [24].

What-If-Tool:

In 2021, Google's "What-If Tool" (WIT) introduced a visual interface for exploring and analyzing the behaviours of trained machine learning (ML) models, minimizing the need for extensive coding. WIT can easily work with platforms like Jupyter, Colaboratory, Cloud AI Notebooks, and TensorBoard. It supports various ML problem types, including binary classification, multi-class classification, and regression, and accommodates diverse data formats such as tabular, image, and text. This flexibility makes WIT a powerful and versatile tool for understanding model behaviours across various data types and problem categories, ultimately enhancing interpretability and decision-making in ML workflows. Furthermore, WIT

Table 5.1 Platform of XAI tools

Tools-name	Developer	Purpose	Specifications	Platform
AI fairness 360[1]	IBM	Pre- and post-modelling	Reduces bias in datasets and models	Python and R
What-If-Tool[2]	Google	Pre- and post-modelling	Examines dataset characteristics and model behaviour	Jupyter and cloud AI
Skater[3]	Oracle	Post-modelling	Facilitate the interpretation of opaque box models	Python
H_2O platform[4]	$H_2$0ai	Post-modelling	Provides a toolkit for post-hoc explainability	AutoML
Model interpretability[5]	Microsoft	Pre- and post modelling	Displays feature importance for the model and Identifies patterns in data	Interactive GUI
ELI5[6]	MIT	Post-modelling	AI model visualization and debugging	Python
Distill[7]	IISC	Post-modelling	Feature interpretation and attribution	Unified interface

Source links:
[1]https://aif360.res.ibm.com/
[2]https://pair-code.github.io/what-if-tool/
[3]https://pypi.org/project/skater/
[4]https://h2o.ai/platform/ai-cloud/
[5]https://interpret.ml/
[6]https://eli5.readthedocs.io/en/latest/
[7]https://distill.pub/

enables the analysis of both model behaviours and data during the pre-modelling and post-modelling stages [25].

Skater:

In 2021, Oracle introduced Skater, a Python library designed to analyze the behaviours of trained models at both global and local levels. Global analysis involves drawing inferences across an entire dataset, while local analysis focuses on the predictions for individual samples. Skater's ability to provide both global and local interpretability empowers users with detailed insights into model behaviours, enabling a comprehensive understanding of system decisions across various contexts and datasets. Additionally, the platform simplifies post-modelling analysis and supports the demystification of black-box models [26].

H_2O platform:

In 2017, H_2O.ai launched the H_2O platform [27], designed to simplify and accelerate the creation and deployment of AI systems across different business applications. By abstracting the technical complexities of AI, it enables users to build AI-powered solutions without requiring coding skills. This user-friendly approach empowers domain experts and business stakeholders to effectively leverage AI, fostering seamless collaboration with data scientists and streamlining the development process. Additionally, the platform supports a post-hoc explainability toolkit and white-box modelling with AutoML.

Model interpretability:

In 2021, Microsoft introduced a comprehensive set of tools and frameworks for enhancing the interpretability of machine learning models, aimed at increasing transparency and understanding. Integrated within the Responsible AI dashboard of Microsoft Azure Machine Learning, these tools include both model-specific and model-agnostic explainers, such as SHAP (SHapley Additive exPlanations), which can be applied to various model types, including tree-based and deep learning models. By providing detailed insights into attribute significance, individual predictions, and overall model behaviours, these tools enable users to better understand complex models and ensure they meet ethical and fairness standards. Microsoft's interpretability solutions build trust in AI systems, empowering data scientists, developers, and business stakeholders to make well-informed decisions and support responsible AI practices [28].

Eli5:

The ELI5 library, designed by MIT, is a Python tool designed for visualizing and debugging machine learning (ML) models. It supports various ML frameworks, including Scikit-learn, Keras, LightGBM, and XGBoost. ELI5 offers explanations in multiple formats, such as text, HTML, web dashboards, and JSON, making it versatile and user-friendly. By visualizing decision paths, highlighting important features, and enabling effective debugging, ELI5 simplifies complex models into understandable insights. This helps users validate models, improve transparency, and build trust in AI systems [29].

Distill:

Distill for XAI refers to methods that simplify and clarify complex machine learning models, making their decision-making process interpretable and transparent. The goal is to "distill" the model's behaviours into easy-to-understand explanations without losing its essence. This involves schemes such as visualizations, attribute importance analysis, and breaking down model decisions step by step. By providing clear insights, distillation helps in understanding, debugging, and building trust in AI systems [30].

5.4 XAI Evaluation Schemes

Evaluation metrics play a critical role in assessing XAI tools. A recent review study [31] categorized these metrics into subjective and objective types, highlighting their challenges. The *Objective metrics* focus on quantitative measures such as simplicity, sensitivity, completeness, soundness, stability, robustness, computational cost, post-model evaluation, faithfulness, ROAR, GT-Shapley, perturbation-based metrics, diversity, explanation correctness, confidence, fidelity, representativity, and non-representativeness. These metrics are divided into task- or method-specific metrics, such as those for example-based methods and counterfactual explanations, and model-related metrics like attribution-based evaluation, perturbation methods, and model performance. These approaches are used in various applications, including recommendation systems, COVID-MANet, Convolutional Neural Networks (CNNs), brain-computer interface systems, and bias detection models, ensuring model stability and reliability. The *Subjective metrics*, which rely on human-based evaluations, involve domain experts or randomly selected participants to assess attributes like transparency, trust, effectiveness, efficiency, satisfaction, justifiability, interactivity, user understanding, and human-AI task performance. While subjective metrics are less commonly implemented in real-world scenarios, they are critical for assessing the user experience of AI systems. Establishing formalized definitions of these metrics is essential for advancing XAI and fostering trust in AI technologies.

5.5 XAI Applications in Healthcare

Researchers are actively working to commercialize AI systems and address their black-box nature using Explainable AI (XAI). This approach has the potential to enhance accountability and drive the wider adoption of AI systems in healthcare. Key applications of XAI in this domain include disease diagnosis, classification, and prediction. Approaches like SHAP, LIME, Grad-CAM, and partial dependence plots are widely used in medical fields such as cardiology, oncology, Alzheimer's, fertility, and neurology. These diseases significantly impact human health, and XAI provides valuable insights by identifying the features that influence AI model outputs, directly linking them to patients' health conditions. In this section, we discuss the role of XAI in various branches of medical science, particularly in addressing diseases that have the greatest impact on human health and whose rapid progression can severely undermine human life. This aspect is covered in our first proposal. The second proposal outlines the role of XAI in reproductive science, with a particular focus on fertility.

5.5.1 Proposal 1: XAI and Common Diseases

This discussion focuses on some of the deadliest diseases, including cardiovascular disease, cancer, and Alzheimer's disease. Notably, these conditions often involve interconnected contributions from comorbidities. A summary of the relationship between these diseases and the role of XAI is provided below.

Cardiovascular disease & XAI:

In [32], the D2AFNet method was proposed using a publicly available dataset, achieving high accuracies of 99.49% and 99.28% for two-class and three-class classification tasks, respectively. This model outperformed others in detecting atrial fibrillation, and the attention vector XAI method was employed to ensure explainability. In [33], the XGB algorithm was implemented to diagnose acute coronary syndrome, achieving an AUC of 94%, with the SHAP approach used to identify top risk markers for both men and women. In [34], Photoplethysmography signals were utilized to track diverse aspects of the circulatory system. The proposed model relied on the ResNet architecture, and three XAI techniques—guided saliency, deepSHAP, and integrated gradients—were applied to explain its predictions. In [35], a deep learning model was introduced for heart rhythm classification, with explainability achieved using SHAP and domain-specific concepts. In [36], the authors suggested six predictive models to estimate six clinical traits, such as left atrial size, left atrial volume, left ventricular ejection fraction, functional classification, left ventricular internal diastolic diameter, and left ventricular internal systolic diameter. The predictions for each of these models were explained using SHAP. In [37], a DenseNet-based deep learning model was developed to screen for major congenital heart diseases, achieving a remarkable accuracy of 100%, with Grad-CAM and guided backpropagation used to provide interpretability. In [38], a hybrid classical-quantum transfer learning approach was employed to predict cardiomegaly, achieving an ROC of 93%, with Grad-CAM++ used to explain the model's reliability. In [39], an if–then rule-based system was implemented to provide interpretability for a model using multi-resolution image parameterization, which improved the diagnostic accuracy for coronary artery disease. In [40], a domain knowledge-guided recurrent network was proposed to predict heart failure, with its performance explained through if–then rules. In [41], the authors used heart failure and cataract symptom data to construct a model based on the RNN algorithm, employing attention mechanisms and if–then rules as XAI tools for interpretability. In [42], a deep neural network was proposed for multilabel arrhythmia detection, with dual-level attention mechanisms employed to enhance explainability. In [43], an interpretable knowledge-guided model named KnowRisk was designed to predict heart failure, using attention weights to explain its predictions. In [44], an ensemble model utilizing the VGG19 architecture was proposed to predict myocardial inversion time. Saliency maps were employed to interpret the model's outputs. In [45], a deep learning model built on a 3D U-Net architecture was introduced to calculate left ventricle volume, with a class activation function used to explain its decision-making process. In [46], a CNN model was developed to classify transthyretin amyloidosis, a known cause of heart failure, achieving an AUC of 94%. The interpretability of the model's predictions was enhanced using maximum activation maps. In [47], a correction method was applied to improve the explainability of a deep neural network, enabling it to effectively identify the strongest ECG features. In [48], an interpretable machine learning model employing a parsimony plot was proposed to predict cardiac arrest, with results clearly explained to support understanding. In [49], AI algorithms such as SVM and CNN were utilized to classify cardiac arrhythmia, with expert-enhanced explanations adding clarity to the results. In [50], a deep learning model based on the LSTM architecture was proposed to predict unplanned cardiac surgeries. Attention heatmaps were implemented to explain its decision-making process. In [51], saliency maps were used to interpret a proposed model designed to classify arrhythmias. In [52], an SVM model was developed for diagnosing heart disease, achieving an accuracy of 94.4%. The model's trustworthiness was explained through clinical expertise and adherence to standard guidelines. In [53], a deep learning model was implemented for the assessment of cardiac function, following a conventional clinical workflow. Frame-by-frame 3D-depth map processes under XAI were used to enhance interpretability. In [54], the xEGGNet fine-tuned model was proposed to detect cardiac arrhythmias, with class attention maps applied to assist clinicians by visually interpreting predictions. In [55], a CNN model was utilized to predict drug-induced arrhythmias and diagnose long QT syndrome. The model demonstrated a high AUC value, with its explainability analyzed through occlusion. In [56], a novel neural network framework named Multi-View Multi-Task Network (MuViTaNet) and its fairness variant (F-MuViTaNet) were proposed for cardiac complication risk profiling. Model interpretability was achieved using feature view attention weights. In [57], a DL -based AI algorithm was utilized for pulmonary hypertension (PH) detection, with model interpretability explained using the Grad-CAM tool. In [58], a DL model was implemented for the classification of cardiac arrhythmias. Additionally, the bootstrap LIME (B-LIME) technique was proposed to provide meaningful explanations. Notably, the explanations generated by the B-LIME hybrid model outperformed those provided by LIME. In [59], a diagnostic tool for arrhythmia was developed, and its performance was compared with a physics-based approach. A direct mapping technique was applied to enhance the interpretability of the proposed model. In [60], a neural network-based regression model was introduced to predict cardiac age, using SHAP for interpretability. In [61], a segmentation model called FAUet, integrating U-Net in series, was proposed to evaluate cardiac function, with model explanations provided through Grad-CAM. Similarly, in [62], a CNN architecture was designed to classify heart failure (HF) from X-rays, with interpretability achieved using Grad-CAM. In [63], a CNN-based model is proposed to predict irregular cardiac patterns. This model enhances the understanding of sample arrangements by utilizing XAI tools such as dynamic time warping, mean squared error, and slack. In [63], a deep learning model was designed to uncover the statistical relationship between body surface potentials (BSP) and cardiac activation, effectively distinguishing between ground truth and activation maps. Interpretability was achieved through activation maps, and the model demonstrated high accuracy on simulated data. In [64], a physics-informed DL model was proposed and evaluated against conventional DL methods. A dictionary learning approach was utilized to understand the model's decision-making process. In [65], a deep neural network (DNN) was developed to detect cardiomyopathy, with the global Grad-CAM++ technique providing feature visualization for model interpretation. In [66], a graph neural network (GNN)-based model called EchoGNN was presented to predict ejection fraction, with interpretability analyzed using learned weights. In [67], an efficient and explainable DL-based early warning system was proposed for predicting cardiac arrest (CA). This system, achieving an AUC of 0.85, captured sequences of clinical parameters via a temporal convolutional network and was explained using the deep Taylor decomposition framework. In [68], a CNN model was employed to identify morphological heart abnormalities. The study also introduced an Explainable AI (XAI) framework for ECG classification, leveraging Class Activation Maps (CAM) from Grad-CAM for interpretation. In [69], a DL model aimed at predicting the success of radio-frequency catheter ablation (RFCA) therapy for atrial fibrillation (AF) was developed, using Grad-CAM, occlusion-based maps, and LIME for interpretability. In [70], the Gini index was employed to assess the interpretability of a machine learning model designed to diagnose early HF. In [71], a DL model for ejection fraction classification integrated Concept Activation Vectors (CAVs) for global and local interpretability in cardiac MRI analysis. In [72], a variational mesh autoencoder (VMAE), representing a novel geometric DL approach, was proposed to identify myocardial infarction. The latent space of the VMAE was used as an XAI tool to assess model quality and interpretability. In [73], a DNN for arrhythmia classification utilized post-hoc explanation tools such as SHAP, LIME, and Grad-CAM to enhance model interpretability. In [74], a CNN-based 3-lead ECG classification model, named lightX3ECG, was introduced, with Grad-CAM and SHAP providing explanations. In [75], SHAP was applied to interpret machine learning models predicting atrial fibrillation, with gradient boosting machines (GBM) emerging as the most effective. SHAP also generated detailed risk profiles. In [76], an explainable DL model was developed to detect congenital heart disease. The interpretability of the model was demonstrated using graph chart diagrams to compare visualized regions in normal and abnormal cases. Finally, in [77], a CNN-based model was proposed for assessing HF, utilizing saliency maps, Grad-CAM, and XRAI tools to interpret the model's decisions.

In a recent review article on cardiac science [78], researchers highlighted that a significant number of studies have utilized Explainable Artificial Intelligence (XAI) techniques, as identified through literature-based evaluation. SHAP and Grad-CAM emerged as the most widely used tools, with SHAP applied to datasets like ECG, CMR, and EHR, while Grad-CAM found extensive use in ECG and other types of data. Additionally, methods such as LIME, PDP, and GBM were identified as key areas of interest for researchers investigating cardiac science with XAI.

However, a critical observation was that many studies implementing XAI approaches lacked formal evaluations of the outcomes, underscoring the need for rigorous validation to enhance the reliability and impact of XAI in this domain.

Alzheimer's disease & XAI:

In [21], SpinalNet and CNN models are proposed to predict Alzheimer's disease (AD) classes from MRI images. Additionally, gene expression data is leveraged for AD classification using three machine learning algorithms: KNN, SVC, and XGB. The findings reveal that CNN performs better for prediction tasks, whereas SVC outperforms others in classification. The LIME tool is utilized to identify significant genes responsible for AD. In [79], the proposed 3D CNN model is analyzed using two post-hoc explanation techniques: saliency maps and layerwise relevance propagation.

These methods effectively illustrate the connection between the assigned importance and the distinctive features of PET signal variations. In [80], neural models such as ResNet50, VGG16, and InceptionV3 are explored, with their results analyzed using the LIME framework. The achieved accuracies are 86.68% for VGG16, 82.26% for ResNet50, and 82.04% for InceptionV3. In [81], a novel method is introduced for diagnosing AD and mild cognitive impairment (MCI). The approach is evaluated using SVM, ANN, and CNN, with LIME applied to highlight brain regions linked to AD/MCI onset and progression. In [82], transformer models are tested, with BERT achieving the highest accuracy of 87.50%. An accuracy of 86.25% is also attained under a multi-task learning setup. Interpretability is assessed using LIME. In [83], a CNN model achieves 94.96% accuracy, with the LIME algorithm providing visual explanations for the model's predictions. In [84], a Random Forest (RF) model is proposed for AD detection, and SHAP is employed to interpret the model's decisions. In [85], an RF-based threefold classification model is implemented, with SHAP explaining the model's viability. In [86], three machine learning classifiers—XGB, SVM, and RF—are deployed, with the SHAP framework providing interpretability. In [87], two ML algorithms are implemented, and the SHAP framework is used for interpreting their performance. In [88], an XGB classifier is developed, with model interpretability provided by the SHAP framework. In [89], four ML classifiers—LR, RF, XGB, and another RF—are applied. Of these, XGB performs best with a ROC value of 0.52 and an accuracy of 80.7%. Model interpretability is explained using SHAP. In [90], a new framework called RS-SSAS is designed for small sample sizes. Random Seeds, SVM-Smote, and RF algorithms are applied, and SHAP facilitates model interpretation. In [91], the SHAP explainer is used to evaluate a proposed SVC-based model, which is compared to DT, LGBM, and RF. In [92], a transfer learning-based framework is introduced, achieving 87% accuracy, with model decisions explained via SHAP. In [93], a CNN architecture attains a 99.9% accuracy rate, with SHAP enhancing the model's interpretability. In [94], a 3D CNN framework coupled with a BRNN model achieves 96% accuracy, with guided Grad-CAM providing model explanations. In [95], five ML algorithms—RF, Bagging, ADA, NB, and XGB—are analyzed using the SHAP XAI framework, showing improved accuracy across models. In [96], a robust Explainable AI model based on deep learning is introduced, with SHAP ensuring interpretability. In [97], SHAP and LIME tools are applied to interpret a voting classifier model that achieves 97.6% accuracy.

In addition to research articles, numerous review papers have focused on the application of XAI in AD studies. A recent study [98] highlighted how XAI tools offer detailed insights into the factors underlying the clinical diagnosis of AD. The study reviewed approximately 85 XAI models, analyzing their datasets, input types, and various AI methodologies, including ML and DL. Among ML tools, XGB emerged as the most effective, while CNNs were favoured within the DL framework. Widely used XAI tools include SHAP, LIME, Grad-CAM, saliency maps, and layerwise relevance propagation (LRP). In the DL context, tools like OCC, 3D CAM, and 3D UCM are commonly utilized, whereas SHAP stands out as the most versatile XAI tool in ML-based frameworks. A separate study [99] discussed the current applications and frameworks of XAI in AD. It introduced a theoretically designed interpretability framework called "Feature Augmented," which remains unexplored due to the limited availability of XAI-specific datasets for AD. Among the commonly used datasets, MRI stands out as the most prevalent, supporting both model-agnostic and model-specific applications of XAI.

Thus, the growing adoption of XAI frameworks in healthcare, particularly for predictive applications, has been instrumental in building trust and confidence within the medical community, reinforcing the credibility of AI-driven approaches for diagnosing Alzheimer's disease.

Cancer disease & XAI:

In [100], a deep learning-based Explainable AI (XAI) model, known as HSCNN, is utilized for lung cancer identification, with an ad-hoc explanation provided using the Explainable Deep Hierarchical Semantic CNN. Similarly, in [101], the SISC architecture is implemented for lung cancer detection, accompanied by an ad-hoc explanation generated through the SISC method. In [102], a deep CNN is applied to detect breast cancer, with the Grad-CAM tool employed for post-hoc model interpretation. Likewise, in [103], a Bayesian neural network is used for brain cancer detection, and model explanations are performed using Grad-CAM. In [104], multimodal mult-label CNNs are employed for prostate cancer detection, with the CAM (Class Activation Map) technique used to interpret the model. In [105], Grad-CAM and saliency maps are integrated to explain an AI model based on the VGGNet architecture. Additionally, in [106], a 20-layer deep residual CNN model is developed for lung cancer diagnosis, interpreted using Grad-CAM. For liver cancer detection, [107] introduces a CNN-based deep learning system, where saliency maps explain the model, and [108] applies the CAM tool for a similar task. In [109], a deep CNN ensemble method identifies breast cancer, and integrated gradients are used for model interpretation. In [110], a capsule network architecture is adopted for breast cancer detection. In contrast, [111] applies the X-Caps method for lung cancer detection, presenting an ad-hoc explanation. Brain cancer diagnosis is addressed in [112] with an explainable model, also providing an ad-hoc explanation. In [113], an AI model for lung cancer detection uses the supervised iterative descent method for interpretability. For breast cancer detection, [114] employs a U-Net transfer learning model with the SHAP XAI tool to assess feature importance. A hybrid model combining XGB and CNN is implemented for lung cancer detection in [115], where the SHAP method explains the proposed DeepXplainer model. In [116], an XGB classifier predicts breast cancer, with SHAP identifying relevant variables and their importance. In [117], an XAI model achieves 97.72% accuracy in cancer image classification. Breast cancer detection is addressed in [118] using the KNN algorithm, with model interpretation handled by LIME. An explainable XGB model is applied in [119] for lung cancer prediction, where SHAP is used for interpretation. In [120], a Faster R-CNN Feature Pyramid Network (FPN) combined with deep learning is used for oral cancer classification and detection, explained via heat maps.

Significant research has been published on cancer applications, with XAI emerging as a key focus area. This analysis emphasizes recent studies, complemented by numerous review articles covering skin, breast, and lung cancers. For example, Hauser et sl. [121] reviews 37 articles exclusively on XAI applications in skin cancer, with most studies employing pretrained DNNs for classification tasks. In [122], a detailed review explores XAI applications for breast cancer detection and prediction, summarizing 30 articles and listing popular machine learning (ML) and deep learning (DL) algorithms. The study also visualizes XAI growth trends using a bubble graph. In [123], a review of AI and XAI-based breast cancer detection tools examines various imaging modalities, highlighting cost-to-accuracy trade-offs across four commonly used modalities.

Moreover, highlighting the urgent need for effective prevention to build a sustainable, disease-free society. XAI or interpretable models play a crucial role in advancing cancer research by enabling early detection and diagnosis. These models enhance transparency in decision-making, helping to identify critical features and foster trust in AI-based predictions. Integrating XAI into cancer detection methods represents a significant step toward improving outcomes, facilitating early intervention, and ultimately supporting cancer prevention efforts.

5.5.2 Proposal 2: XAI and Reproductive Science

Reproductive science is a rapidly advancing field that encompasses a wide range of disciplines, including reproductive biology, medicine, obstetrics, gynaecology, maternal–fetal medicine, fertility and infertility, and contraception. The increasing volume of medical research published in this area reflects its dynamic and evolving nature. This proposal focuses on key application areas within reproductive science where the interpretability of AI models plays a critical role. Male infertility has become a global concern, and AI has shown significant potential in predicting fertility issues at an early stage. In [124], researchers employed seven industry-standard AI algorithms to predict male fertility, achieving varying levels of accuracy. The study emphasized model interpretability, using SHAP to explain the decision-making process of each algorithm. In [125], an Explainable AI model was developed using the XGB algorithm, with its interpretability achieved through SHAP and LIME tools. This approach enabled accurate predictions of male fertility status. Similarly, [126] introduced an explainable machine learning model to predict reproductive outcomes following frozen embryo transfer. The use of a SHAP summary plot highlighted the influence of individual features on the predictive model. A review in [127] explored the transition in embryo selection methodologies, moving from opaque black-box models to more transparent glass-box systems. This review analyzed 13 morphology-based embryo decision support systems and emphasized the interpretability and usability of glass-box models, which address the growing challenges associated with black-box approaches. The need for XAI in female fertility analysis is discussed in [128], highlighting its role in fostering trust and acceptance of AI models within the domain. In [129], the significance of predictive modelling for the future of reproductive medicine is examined, with explainability identified as one of the primary challenges in the commercialization of AI models in this field. In [130], an XAI model is developed to identify follicles and improve outcomes in in vitro fertilization (IVF). The study highlights the significant influence of follicle size on increasing live birth rates. The model, built using gradient boosting regression trees, is interpreted through SHAP analysis. In [131], an ensemble XAI approach, incorporating the SHAP tool, is employed to accurately determine follicle sizes. In [132], a machine learning-based interpretable AI model is introduced for embryo selection, enhancing decision-making in IVF. In [133], a DL algorithm is designed for embryo assessment. Explainable AI techniques, such as Grad-CAM and LIME, are applied to identify key features in embryo images related to specific embryonic cleavage stages. In [134], five black box machine learning models, including bagging classifier, random forest, XGB, CatBoost, and extra trees, are applied to predict the risk of pregnancy termination using 338,904 instances and 18 features. Explainable AI tools such as SHAP, Eli5, and LIME are employed to identify the most significant features contributing to this risk. Among these models, the random forest achieved the highest accuracy. The analysis reveals that wealth index, current work experience, source of drinking water, sex of the household head, education level, and marital status are the most influential factors, providing valuable insights into reproductive healthcare in East Africa. In [135], six machine learning models, including RF, linear discriminant analysis (LDA), LR, SVM, ADA, and LGBM, are trained to predict the ploidy status of embryos. Random forest outperformed the other models, achieving an accuracy of 74.9% and an AUC of 0.808. The model's performance was validated using external datasets, with the SHAP tool employed to analyze feature importance, and LIME used to provide prediction probabilities. In [136], a Random Forest (RF) model was employed to predict maternal outcomes, with its interpretability demonstrated using two XAI frameworks: SHAP and LIME. This methodology holds significant potential to improve medical decision-making, offering benefits to both mothers and their children. In [137], an XAI model based on XGB algorithms is developed to predict the risk of maternal health issues. The model employs SHAP and LIME to offer clear explanations of its predictions. In [138], a U-Net architecture is utilized to predict blastocyst formation, with an XAI tool identifying the key factors influencing this process. In [139], seven machine learning algorithms are used to predict unintended pregnancies, with XGB delivering the best performance. SHAP is employed to explain the model's predictions and to identify the primary predictors of unintended pregnancy. In [140], an XAI model utilizing a DL architecture was developed to analyze PCOS, achieving a 97% accuracy. The model's interpretation was provided through SHAP and LIME, with the study highlighting insulin levels as the most significant factor influencing PCOS, followed by the number of follicles in the right ovary (R) and left ovary (L). Study [141] applied a RF model to predict PCOS risk, incorporating the LIME method to assess and interpret the identified risk factors. Similarly, in [142], an XAI model was designed to detect PCOS, utilizing a grey wolf-based feature selection method. This model, which was explained using LIME, achieved an outstanding accuracy of 97.42%. In [143], a unique XAI framework was introduced for PCOS detection, combining three interpretation tools: LIME, SHAP, and ELI5. Additionally, QGraph was used to further analyze the results from the trained models. In [144], another XAI framework was proposed for the early detection of PCOS, with both LIME and SHAP tools applied to interpret the model's predictions. In [145], the XGB ensemble machine learning model was employed to predict PCOS, with SHAP used for global interpretation of the model. Additionally, LIME was utilized to provide local explanations, illustrating the influence of features on the classifier's decisions. In [146], an XAI model was deployed for PCOS detection, with SHAP offering global interpretability for the model.

After reviewing all the articles, it is evident that XAI plays a crucial role in advancing reproductive science, particularly in areas such as IVF, fertility prediction, PCOS detection and maternal health. However, there is a noticeable scarcity of studies employing XAI tools in this domain. While most researchers have relied on traditional machine learning techniques, the datasets used are often limited, especially for male fertility prediction. On the other hand, larger datasets become available when supported by national initiatives. Despite these advancements, the commercialization of AI systems for reproductive healthcare remains restricted, and generalizability across populations remains a challenge. Therefore, integrating XAI into reproductive science emerges as a critical priority to enhance model reliability and broaden its practical applications.

5.6 Conceptual Overview of Case Studies

Case studies underscore the pivotal role of XAI in healthcare, with applications spanning disease diagnosis, prediction, and advancements in reproductive health. XAI is founded on the principles of interpretability and the ability to clarify the decision-making process of AI systems. These features contribute significantly to the commercialization of AI in healthcare. Explanations offered by XAI can also be categorized based on their mode of delivery.

This chapter examines numerous studies on ML, DL, and their applications across various domains. It highlights the range of methodologies and frameworks implemented using XAI tools such as Grad-CAM, SHAP, LIME, LRP, PCR, HAM, SM, OCC, 3D Grad-CAM, GNNE, heatmaps, and decision trees. Common visual aids include waterfall plots, force plots, stacked force plots, mean SHAP plots, and dependence plots.

XAI is closely linked with the concept of feature relevance, which involves assigning specific scores to data attributes to quantify their importance. By providing high-quality explanations, XAI ensures that physicians, as primary stakeholders in healthcare, can confidently interpret AI-driven decisions. The capability of XAI extends beyond analyzing various data types (e.g., tabular data, textual inputs, and images) to processing signals such as ECG, EEG, and PCG. Similarly, XAI has been utilized to analyze one-dimensional biosignals and text data, such as clinical notes.

SHAP is predominantly used in ML models, while Grad-CAM is widely applied in DL models. LIME, on the other hand, is versatile and can be employed in both contexts. These XAI tools differ in their focus: LIME emphasizes local interpretability, whereas SHAP offers insights on both a global and local level. Beyond

SHAP, LIME, Grad-CAM, CAM, heatmaps, and attribution methods, other techniques such as anchors, GraphLIME, LRP, DTD, PDA, TCAV, XGNN, ASV, breakdown analysis, Shapley flow, textual explanations of visual models, integrated gradients, causal models, meaningful perturbations, and X-NeSy have also been introduced to healthcare applications. These methodologies mark a transformative phase in healthcare, emphasizing legitimacy, ethics, and robustness for sustainable, reliable solutions.

However, many researchers have yet to incorporate performance metrics into their XAI models. Most published work prioritizes subjective evaluation methods, highlighting the challenges associated with user-centred assessments. Nevertheless, XAI represents a significant transition toward human-centred, multidisciplinary research. The growing demand for XAI stems from several crucial factors: (a) It verifies that AI models make predictions based on accurate data, (b) It aids in refining AI models' hyperparameters, and (c) It facilitates comparisons of AI models used across similar studies with varying datasets.

In healthcare, challenges like dataset uncertainty are particularly evident in reproductive science. Additionally, the diversity of applications, datasets, and model types complicates consistent evaluation of AI models, making XAI-driven explanations more critical. Despite its potential, many XAI tools remain underexplored in reproductive science, where they are urgently needed. Potential applications include male fertility analysis, IVF success rate prediction, improved embryo and gamete selection, evaluation prediction, and optimization of medications.

Currently, a lack of transparency hinders the widespread commercialization of AI models. To foster rapid innovation in healthcare and achieve improved clinical outcomes in reproductive science, integrating XAI into future advancements is not just beneficial—it is imperative.

5.7 Conclusion

The transformative impact of XAI in healthcare, including reproductive science, is clear. Tools like SHAP simplify model explanations by highlighting critical clinical features, with applications such as male fertility detection, PCOS diagnosis, and embryos selection. Frameworks like LIME and Grad-CAM complement SHAP, particularly in deep learning models, enabling insights into advanced methods like graph neural networks and reinforcement learning. The XAI's human-centred approach helps patients and medical professionals interpret AI outputs, driving trust and transparency. Hence, collaboration between data scientists and healthcare experts is essential to develop reliable XAI applications, enhancing medical practices, improving patient outcomes, and fostering innovation in treatments and diagnostics.

References

1. Lee, C. H., Wang, C., Fan, X., Li, F., & Chen, C. H. (2023). Artificial intelligence-enabled digital transformation in elderly healthcare field: Scoping review. *Advanced Engineering Informatics, 55*, Article 101874.
2. Arrieta, A. B., Díaz-Rodríguez, N., Del Ser, J., Bennetot, A., Tabik, S., Barbado, A., Garcia, S., Gil-Lopez, S., Molina, D., Benjamins, R., Chatila, R., & Herrera, F. (2020). Explainable artificial intelligence (XAI): Concepts, taxonomies, opportunities and challenges toward responsible AI. *Information Fusion, 58*, 82–115.
3. Schoonderwoerd, T. A., Jorritsma, W., Neerincx, M. A., & Van Den Bosch, K. (2021). Human-centered XAI: Developing design patterns for explanations of clinical decision support systems. *International Journal of Human-Computer Studies, 154*, Article 102684.
4. Antoniadi, A. M., Du, Y., Guendouz, Y., Wei, L., Mazo, C., Becker, B. A., & Mooney, C. (2021). Current challenges and future opportunities for XAI in machine learning-based clinical decision support systems: A systematic review. *Applied Sciences, 11*(11), 5088.
5. Pinto-Coelho, L. (2023). How artificial intelligence is shaping medical imaging technology: A survey of innovations and applications. *Bioengineering (Basel, Switzerland), 10*(12), 1435. https://doi.org/10.3390/bioengineering10121435
6. Seo, H., Badiei Khuzani, M., Vasudevan, V., Huang, C., Ren, H., Xiao, R., Jia, X., & Xing, L. (2020). Machine learning techniques for biomedical image segmentation: An overview of technical aspects and introduction to state-of-art applications. *Medical Physics, 47*(5), e148–e167. https://doi.org/10.1002/mp.13649
7. Hassija, V., Chamola, V., Mahapatra, A., Singal, A., Goel, D., Huang, K., Scardapane, S., Spinelli, I., Mahmud, M., & Hussain, A. (2024). Interpreting black-box models: A review on explainable artificial intelligence. *Cognitive Computation, 16*(1), 45–74.
8. Hendrickson, R. G. (1984). A survey of sensitivity analysis methodology.
9. Mienye, I. D., Obaido, G., Jere, N., Mienye, E., Aruleba, K., Emmanuel, I. D., & Ogbuokiri, B. (2024). A survey of explainable artificial intelligence in healthcare: Concepts, applications, and challenges. *Informatics in Medicine Unlocked*, 101587.
10. Weber, L., Lapuschkin, S., Binder, A., & Samek, W. (2023). Beyond explaining: Opportunities and challenges of XAI-based model improvement. *Information Fusion, 92*, 154–176.
11. Sadeghi, Z., Alizadehsani, R., CIFCI, M. A., Kausar, S., Rehman, R., Mahanta, P., & Pardalos, P. M., et al. (2024). A review of explainable artificial. In S. Bach, A. Binder, G. Montavon, F. Klauschen, K. R. Müller, & W. Samek, (2015). On pixel-wise explanations for non-linear classifier decisions by layer-wise relevance propagation. *PloS one, 10*(7), e0130140. Intelligence in healthcare. *Computers and Electrical Engineering, 118*, 109370.
12. Linardatos, P., Papastefanopoulos, V., & Kotsiantis, S. (2020). Explainable Ai: A review of machine learning interpretability methods. *Entropy, 23*(1), 18.
13. Habib, G., & Qureshi, S. (2022). Optimization and acceleration of a review of explainable artificial intelligence in healthcare. Convolutional neural networks: A survey. *Journal of King Saud University-Computer and Information Sciences, 34*(7), 4244–4268.
14. Floridi, L. (2021). Establishing the rules for building trustworthy AI. *Ethics, Governance, and Policies in Artificial Intelligence*, 41–45.
15. Shams Khoozani, Z., Sabri, A. Q. M., Seng, W. C., Seera, M., & Eg, K. Y. (2024). Navigating the landscape of concept-supported XAI: Challenges, innovations, and future directions. *Multimedia Tools and Applications*, 1–51.
16. Bach, S., Binder, A., Montavon, G., Klauschen, F., Müller, K. R., & Samek, W. (2015). On pixel-wise explanations for non-linear classifier decisions by layer-wise relevance propagation. *PLoS ONE, 10*(7), Article e0130140.
17. Selvaraju, R. R., Cogswell, M., Das, A., Vedantam, R., Parikh, D., & Batra, D. (2017). Grad-cam: Visual explanations from deep networks via gradient-based localization. In *Proceedings of the IEEE international conference on computer vision* (pp. 618–626).

18. Cirqueira, D., Nedbal, D., Helfert, M., & Bezbradica, M. (2020, August). Scenario-based requirements elicitation for user-centric explainable AI: A case in fraud detection. In *International cross-domain conference for machine learning and knowledge extraction* (pp. 321–341). Springer International Publishing.
19. Alicioglu, G., & Sun, B. (2022). A survey of visual analytics for explainable artificial intelligence methods. *Computers & Graphics, 102*, 502–520.
20. Kim, B., Wattenberg, M., Gilmer, J., Cai, C., Wexler, J., & Viegas, F. (2018, July). Interpretability beyond feature attribution: Quantitative testing with concept activation vectors (tcav). In *International conference on machine learning* (pp. 2668–2677). PMLR.
21. Kamal, M. S., Northcote, A., Chowdhury, L., Dey, N., Crespo, R. G., & Herrera-Viedma, E. (2021). Alzheimer's patient analysis using image and gene expression data and explainable-AI to present associated genes. *IEEE Transactions on Instrumentation and Measurement, 70*, 1–7.
22. Biffi, C., Cerrolaza, J. J., Tarroni, G., Bai, W., De Marvao, A., Oktay, O., Ledig, C., Le Folgoc, L., Kamnitsas, K., Doumou, G., Duan, J., Prasad, S. K., Cook, S. A., O'Regan, D. P., & Rueckert, D. (2020). Explainable anatomical shape analysis through deep hierarchical generative models. *IEEE Transactions on Medical Imaging, 39*(6), 2088–2099.
23. Carson, D. L., & Botha, F. C. (2000). Preliminary analysis of expressed sequence tags for sugarcane. *Crop Science, 40*(6), 1769–1779.
24. Bellamy, R. K., Dey, K., Hind, M., Hoffman, S. C., Houde, S., Kannan, K., Natesan Ramamurthy, K., Richards, J., Saha, D., Sattigeri, P., Singh, M., Varshney, K. R., & Zhang, Y. (2019). AI Fairness 360: An extensible toolkit for detecting and mitigating algorithmic bias. *IBM Journal of Research and Development, 63*(4/5), 4–1.
25. Wexler, J., Pushkarna, M., Bolukbasi, T., Wattenberg, M., Viégas, F., & Wilson, J. (2019). The what-if tool: Interactive probing of machine learning models. *IEEE Transactions on Visualization and Computer Graphics, 26*(1), 56–65.
26. Zhang, J. D., Xue, C., Kolachalama, V. B., & Donald, W. A. (2023). Interpretable machine learning on metabolomics data reveals biomarkers for parkinson's disease. *ACS Central Science, 9*(5), 1035–1045.
27. Kaplan, A., & Haenlein, M. (2019). Siri, Siri, in my hand: Who's the fairest in the land? On the interpretations, illustrations, and implications of artificial intelligence. *Business Horizons, 62*(1), 15–25.
28. Kaur, H., Nori, H., Jenkins, S., Caruana, R., Wallach, H., & Wortman Vaughan, J. (2020, April). Interpreting interpretability: understanding data scientists' use of interpretability tools for machine learning. In *Proceedings of the 2020 CHI conference on human factors in computing systems* (pp. 1–14).
29. Kawakura, S., Hirafuji, M., Ninomiya, S., & Shibasaki, R. (2022). Adaptations of explainable artificial intelligence (XAI) to agricultural data models with ELI5, PDPbox, and skater using diverse agricultural worker data. *European Journal of Artificial Intelligence and Machine Learning, 1*(3), 27–34.
30. Zhang, Y., Tiňo, P., Leonardis, A., & Tang, K. (2021). A survey on neural network interpretability. *IEEE Transactions on Emerging Topics in Computational Intelligence, 5*(5), 726–742.
31. Coroama, L., & Groza, A. (2022, September). Evaluation metrics in explainable artificial intelligence (XAI). In *International conference on advanced research in technologies, information, innovation and sustainability* (pp. 401–413). Springer Nature Switzerland.
32. Zhang, P., Ma, C., Song, F., Sun, Y., Feng, Y., He, Y., Zhang, T., & Zhang, G. (2023). D2AFNet: A dual-domain attention cascade network for accurate and interpretable atrial fibrillation detection. *Biomedical Signal Processing and Control, 82*, 104615.
33. Vazquez, B., Fuentes-Pineda, G., Garcia, F., Borrayo, G., & Prohias, J. (2021). Risk markers by sex for in-hospital mortality in patients with acute coronary syndrome: A machine learning approach. *Informatics in Medicine Unlocked, 27*, Article 100791.
34. Zhang, O., Ding, C., Pereira, T., Xiao, R., Gadhoumi, K., Meisel, K., Lee, R. J., Chen, Y., & Hu, X. (2021). Explain ability metrics of deep convolutional networks for photo plethysmography quality assessment. *IEEE Access, 9*, 29736–29745.

35. Sangroya, A., Jain, S., Vig, L., Anantaram, C., Ukil, A., & Khandelwal, S. (2022, May). Generating conceptual explanations for DL based ECG classification model. In *The international FLAIRS conference proceedings* (vol. 35).
36. Pičulin, M., Smole, T., Žunkovič, B., Kokalj, E., Robnik-Šikonja, M., Kukar, M., Fotiadis, D. I., Pezoulas, V. C., Tachos, N. S., Barlocco, F., Mazzarotto, F., … Bosnić, Z. (2022). Disease progression of hypertrophic cardiomyopathy: modeling using machine learning. *JMIR Medical Informatics, 10*(2), e30483.
37. Nurmaini, S., Partan, R. U., Bernolian, N., Sapitri, A. I., Tutuko, B., Rachmatullah, M. N., Darmawahyuni, A., Firdaus, F., & Mose, J. C. (2022). Deep learning for improving the effectiveness of routine prenatal screening for major congenital heart diseases. *Journal of Clinical Medicine, 11*(21), 6454.
38. Decoodt, P., Liang, T. J., Bopardikar, S., Santhanam, H., Eyembe, A., Garcia-Zapirain, B., & Sierra-Sosa, D. (2023). Hybrid classical–quantum transfer learning for cardiomegaly detection in chest x-rays. *Journal of Imaging, 9*(7), 128.
39. Kukar, M., Kononenko, I., & Grošelj, C. (2011). Modern parameterization and explanation techniques in diagnostic decision support system: A case study in diagnostics of coronary artery disease. *Artificial Intelligence in Medicine, 52*(2), 77–90.
40. Li, R., Yin, C., Yang, S., Qian, B., & Zhang, P. (2020). Marrying medical domain knowledge with deep learning on electronic health records: A deep visual analytics approach. *Journal of Medical Internet Research, 22*(9), Article e20645.
41. Kwon, B. C., Choi, M. J., Kim, J. T., Choi, E., Kim, Y. B., Kwon, S., Sun, J., & Choo, J. (2018). Retainvis: Visual analytics with interpretable and interactive recurrent neural networks on electronic medical records. *IEEE Transactions on Visualization and Computer Graphics, 25*(1), 299–309.
42. Jin, Y., Liu, J., Liu, Y., Qin, C., Li, Z., Xiao, D., Zhao, L., & Liu, C. (2021). A novel interpretable method based on dual-level attentional deep neural network for actual multilabel arrhythmia detection. *IEEE Transactions on Instrumentation and Measurement, 71*, 1–11.
43. Zhang, X., Qian, B., Li, Y., Yin, C., Wang, X., & Zheng, Q. (2019, November). KnowRisk: An interpretable knowledge-guided model for disease risk prediction. In *2019 IEEE international conference on data mining (ICDM)* (pp. 1492–1497). IEEE.
44. Bahrami, N., Retson, T., Blansit, K., Wang, K., & Hsiao, A. (2019). Automated selection of myocardial inversion time with a convolutional neural network: Spatial temporal ensemble myocardium inversion network (STEMI-NET). *Magnetic Resonance in Medicine, 81*(5), 3283–3291.
45. Pérez-Pelegrí, M., Monmeneu, J. V., López-Lereu, M. P., Pérez-Pelegrí, L., Maceira, A. M., Bodí, V., & Moratal, D. (2021). Automatic left ventricle volume calculation with explainability through a deep learning weak-supervision methodology. *Computer Methods and Programs in Biomedicine, 208*, Article 106275.
46. Halme, H. L., Ihalainen, T., Suomalainen, O., Loimaala, A., Mätzke, S., Uusitalo, V., Sipila, O., & Hippeläinen, E. (2022). Convolutional neural networks for detection of transthyretin amyloidosis in 2D scintigraphy images. *EJNMMI Research, 12*(1), 27.
47. Attia, Z. I., Lerman, G., & Friedman, P. A. (2021). Deep neural networks learn by using human-selected electrocardiogram features and novel features. *European Heart Journal-Digital Health, 2*(3), 446–455.
48. Wong, X. Y., Ang, Y. K., Li, K., Chin, Y. H., Lam, S. S. W., Tan, K. B. K., Chua, M. C. H., Ong, M. E. H., Liu, N., Pourghaderi, A. R., Ho, A. F. W., & PAROS Singapore Investigators. (2022). Development and validation of the SARICA score to predict survival after return of spontaneous circulation in out of hospital cardiac arrest using an interpretable machine learning framework. *Resuscitation, 170*, 126–133.
49. Sager, S., Bernhardt, F., Kehrle, F., Merkert, M., Potschka, A., Meder, B., Katus, H., & Scholz, E. (2021). Expert-enhanced machine learning for cardiac arrhythmia classification. *PLoS ONE, 16*(12), Article e0261571.
50. Hur, C., Wi, J., & Kim, Y. (2020). Facilitating the development of deep learning models with visual analytics for electronic health records. *International Journal of Environmental Research and Public Health, 17*(22), 8303.

51. Jones, Y., Deligianni, F., & Dalton, J. (2020, October). Improving ECG classification interpretability using saliency maps. In *2020 IEEE 20th international conference on bioinformatics and bioengineering (BIBE)* (pp. 675–682). IEEE.
52. Meng, J., & Xing, R. (2022). Inside the "black box": Embedding clinical knowledge in data-driven machine learning for heart disease diagnosis. *Cardiovascular Digital Health Journal, 3*(6), 276–288.
53. Duffy, G., Jain, I., He, B., & Ouyang, D. (2021). Interpretable deep learning prediction of 3d assessment of cardiac function. In *Pacific symposium on biocomputing 2022* (pp. 231–241).
54. Yoo, J., Jun, T. J., & Kim, Y. H. (2021). XECGNet: Fine-tuning attention map within convolutional neural network to improve detection and explainability of concurrent cardiac arrhythmias. *Computer Methods and Programs in Biomedicine, 208*, Article 106281.
55. Prifti, E., Fall, A., Davogustto, G., Pulini, A., Denjoy, I., Funck-Brentano, C., Khan, Y., Durand-Salmon, A., Badilini, F., Wells, Q. S., Leenhardt, A., … Salem, J. E. (2021). Deep learning analysis of electrocardiogram for risk prediction of drug-induced arrhythmias and diagnosis of long QT syndrome. *European Heart Journal, 42*(38), 3948–3961.
56. Pham, T. H., Yin, C., Mehta, L., Zhang, X., & Zhang, P. (2023). A fair and interpretable network for clinical risk prediction: A regularized multi-view multi-task learning approach. *Knowledge and Information Systems, 65*(4), 1487–1521.
57. Kwon, J. M., Kim, K. H., Medina-Inojosa, J., Jeon, K. H., Park, J., & Oh, B. H. (2020). Artificial intelligence for early prediction of pulmonary hypertension using electrocardiography. *The Journal of Heart and Lung Transplantation, 39*(8), 805–814.
58. Abdullah, T. A., Zahid, M. S. M., Ali, W., & Hassan, S. U. (2023). B-LIME: An improvement of LIME for interpretable deep learning classification of cardiac arrhythmia from ECG signals. *Processes, 11*(2), 595.
59. Karoui, A., Bendahmane, M., & Zemzemi, N. (2021). Cardiac activation maps reconstruction: A comparative study between data-driven and physics-based methods. *Frontiers in Physiology, 12*, Article 686136.
60. van der Wall, H. E., Hassing, G. J., Doll, R. J., van Westen, G. J., Cohen, A. F., Selder, J. L., Kemme, M., Burggraaf, M., & Gal, P. (2022). Cardiac age detected by machine learning applied to the surface ECG of healthy subjects: Creation of a benchmark. *Journal of Electrocardiology, 72*, 49–55.
61. Wang, Y., Chen, W., Tang, T., Xie, W., Jiang, Y., Zhang, H., Zhou, X., & Yuan, K. (2022). Cardiac segmentation method based on domain knowledge. *Ultrasonic Imaging, 44*(2–3), 105–117.
62. Tsuji, T., Hirata, Y., Kusunose, K., Sata, M., Kumagai, S., Shiraishi, K., & Kotoku, J. I. (2023). Classification of chest X-ray images by incorporation of medical domain knowledge into operation branch networks. *BMC Medical Imaging, 23*(1), 62.
63. Dakshit, S., Maweu, B. M., Dakshit, S., & Prabhakaran, B. (2022, June). Core-set selection using metrics-based explanations (CSUME) for multiclass ECG. In *2022 IEEE 10th international conference on healthcare informatics (ICHI)* (pp. 217–225). IEEE.
64. Kofler, A., Pali, M. C., Schaeffter, T., & Kolbitsch, C. (2023). Deep supervised dictionary learning by algorithm unrolling—Application to fast 2D dynamic MR image reconstruction. *Medical Physics, 50*(5), 2939–2960.
65. van de Leur, R. R., Taha, K., Bos, M. N., van der Heijden, J. F., Gupta, D., Cramer, M. J., Hassink, R. J., van der Harst, P., Doevendans, P. A., Asselbergs, F. W., & van Es, R. (2021). Discovering and visualizing disease-specific electrocardiogram features using deep learning: Proof-of-concept in phospholamban gene mutation carriers. *Circulation: Arrhythmia and Electrophysiology, 14*(2), e009056.
66. Mokhtari, M., Tsang, T., Abolmaesumi, P., & Liao, R. (2022, September). EchoGNN: explainable ejection fraction estimation with graph neural networks. In *International conference on medical image computing and computer-assisted intervention* (pp. 360–369). Springer Nature Switzerland.
67. Tang, Q., Cen, X., & Pan, C. (2022). Explainable and efficient deep early warning system for cardiac arrest prediction from electronic health records. *Mathematical Biosciences and Engineering, 19*, 9825–9841.

68. Ganeshkumar, M., Ravi, V., Sowmya, V., Gopalakrishnan, E. A., & Soman, K. P. (2021). Explainable deep learning-based approach for multilabel classification of electrocardiogram. *IEEE Transactions on Engineering Management, 70*(8), 2787–2799.
69. Ogbomo-Harmitt, S., Muffoletto, M., Zeidan, A., Qureshi, A., King, A. P., & Aslanidi, O. (2023). Exploring interpretability in deep learning prediction of successful ablation therapy for atrial fibrillation. *Frontiers in Physiology, 14*, 1054401.
70. Panicacci, S., Donati, M., Fanucci, L., Bellini, I., Profili, F., & Francesconi, P. (2019, June). Exploring machine learning algorithms to identify heart failure patients: the tuscany region case study. In *2019 IEEE 32nd international symposium on computer-based medical systems (CBMS)* (pp. 417–422). IEEE.
71. Clough, J. R., Oksuz, I., Puyol-Antón, E., Ruijsink, B., King, A. P., & Schnabel, J. A. (2019, October). Global and local interpretability for cardiac MRI classification. In *International conference on medical image computing and computer-assisted intervention* (pp. 656–664). Springer International Publishing.
72. Beetz, M., Corral Acero, J., Banerjee, A., Eitel, I., Zacur, E., Lange, T., Stiermaier, T., Evertz, R., Backhaus, S. J., Thiele, H., Bueno-Orovio, A., Lamata, P., Schuster, A. & Grau, V. (2022). Interpretable cardiac anatomy modeling using variational mesh autoencoders. *Frontiers in Cardiovascular Medicine, 9*, 983868.
73. Singh, P., & Sharma, A. (2022). Interpretation and classification of arrhythmia using deep convolutional network. *IEEE Transactions on Instrumentation and Measurement, 71*, 1–12.
74. Le, K. H., Pham, H. H., Nguyen, T. B., Nguyen, T. A., Thanh, T. N., & Do, C. D. (2023). Lightx3ecg: A lightweight and explainable deep learning system for 3-lead electrocardiogram classification. *Biomedical Signal Processing and Control, 85*, Article 104963.
75. Karri, R., Kawai, A., Thong, Y. J., Ramson, D. M., Perry, L. A., Segal, R., Smith, J. A., & Penny-Dimri, J. C. (2021). Machine learning outperforms existing clinical scoring tools in the prediction of postoperative atrial fibrillation during intensive care unit admission after cardiac surgery. *Heart, Lung and Circulation, 30*(12), 1929–1937.
76. Sakai, A., Komatsu, M., Komatsu, R., Matsuoka, R., Yasutomi, S., Dozen, A., Shozu, K., Arakaki, T., Machino, H., Asada, K., Kaneko, S., Sekizawa, A., & Hamamoto, R. (2022). Medical professional enhancement using explainable artificial intelligence in fetal cardiac ultrasound screening. *Biomedicines, 10*(3), 551.
77. Huynh, J., Masoudi, S., Noorbakhsh, A., Mahmoodi, A., Kligerman, S., Yen, A., Jacobs, K., Hahn, L., Hasenstab, K., Pazzani, M., & Hsiao, A. (2022). Deep learning radiographic assessment of pulmonary edema: Optimizing clinical performance, training with serum biomarkers. *IEEE Access, 10*, 48577–48588.
78. Salih, A. M., Galazzo, I. B., Gkontra, P., Rauseo, E., Lee, A. M., Lekadir, K., Radeva, P., Petersen, S. E., & Menegaz, G. (2024). A review of evaluation approaches for explainable AI with applications in cardiology. *Artificial Intelligence Review, 57*(9), 240.
79. De Santi, L. A., Pasini, E., Santarelli, M. F., Genovesi, D., & Positano, V. (2023). An explainable convolutional neural network for the early diagnosis of Alzheimer's disease from 18F-FDG PET. *Journal of Digital Imaging, 36*(1), 189–203.
80. Shad, H. A., Rahman, Q. A., Asad, N. B., Bakshi, A. Z., Mursalin, S. F., Reza, M. T., & Parvez, M. Z. (2021, December). Exploring Alzheimer's disease prediction with XAI in various neural network models. In *TENCON 2021–2021 IEEE region 10 conference (TENCON)* (pp. 720–725). IEEE.
81. Sidulova, M., Nehme, N., & Park, C. H. (2021, October). Towards explainable image analysis for Alzheimer's disease and mild cognitive impairment diagnosis. In *2021 IEEE applied imagery pattern recognition workshop (AIPR)* (pp. 1–6). IEEE.
82. Ilias, L., & Askounis, D. (2022). Interpretability of deep neural networks used for the diagnosis of Alzheimer's disease. *IEEE Journal of Biomedical and Health Informatics, 26*(8), 4153–4164.
83. Duamwan, L. M., & Bird, J. J. (2023, July). Explainable AI for medical image processing: a study on MRI in Alzheimer's disease. In *Proceedings of the 16th international conference on pervasive technologies related to assistive environments* (pp. 480–484).

84. El-Sappagh, S., Alonso, J. M., Islam, S. R., Sultan, A. M., & Kwak, K. S. (2021). A multilayer multimodal detection and prediction model based on explainable artificial intelligence for Alzheimer's disease. *Scientific Reports, 11*(1), 2660.
85. Bloch, L., Friedrich, C. M., & Alzheimer's Disease Neuroimaging Initiative. (2021). Data analysis with Shapley values for automatic subject selection in Alzheimer's disease data sets using interpretable machine learning. *Alzheimer's Research & Therapy, 13*, 1–30.
86. Hernandez, M., Ramon-Julvez, U., Ferraz, F., & with the ADNI Consortium. (2022). Explainable AI toward understanding the performance of the top three TADPOLE challenge methods in the forecast of Alzheimer's disease diagnosis. *PloS one, 17*(5), e0264695.
87. Lai, Y., Lin, X., Lin, C., Lin, X., Chen, Z., & Zhang, L. (2022). Identification of endoplasmic reticulum stress-associated genes and subtypes for prediction of Alzheimer's disease based on interpretable machine learning. *Frontiers in Pharmacology, 13*, Article 975774.
88. Bogdanovic, B., Eftimov, T., & Simjanoska, M. (2022). In-depth insights into Alzheimer's disease by using explainable machine learning approach. *Scientific Reports, 12*(1), 6508.
89. Chun, M. Y., Park, C. J., Kim, J., Jeong, J. H., Jang, H., Kim, K., & Seo, S. W. (2022). Prediction of conversion to dementia using interpretable machine learning in patients with amnestic mild cognitive impairment. *Frontiers in Aging Neuroscience, 14*, Article 898940.
90. Xu, X., & Yan, X. (2022, August). A convenient and reliable multi-class classification model based on explainable artificial intelligence for Alzheimer's disease. In *2022 IEEE international conference on advances in electrical engineering and computer applications (AEECA)* (pp. 671–675). IEEE. (101).
91. Salih, A., Galazzo, I. B., Cruciani, F., Brusini, L., & Radeva, P. (2022, October). Investigating explainable artificial intelligence for MRI-based classification of dementia: a new stability criterion for explainable methods. In *2022 IEEE international conference on image processing (ICIP)* (pp. 4003–4007). IEEE.
92. Danso, S. O., Zeng, Z., Muniz-Terrera, G., & Ritchie, C. W. (2021). Developing an explainable machine learning-based personalised dementia risk prediction model: A transfer learning approach with ensemble learning algorithms. *Frontiers in Big Data, 4*, Article 613047.
93. Yilmaz, D. (2023, September). Development and evaluation of an explainable diagnostic AI for Alzheimer's disease. In *2023 international conference on artificial intelligence science and applications in industry and society (CAISAIS)* (pp. 1–6). IEEE.
94. Rahim, N., El-Sappagh, S., Ali, S., Muhammad, K., Del Ser, J., & Abuhmed, T. (2023). Prediction of Alzheimer's progression based on multimodal deep-learning-based fusion and visual explainability of time-series data. *Information Fusion, 92*, 363–388.
95. Yi, F., Yang, H., Chen, D., Qin, Y., Han, H., Cui, J., Bai, W., Ma, Y., Zhang, R., & Yu, H. (2023). XGBoost-SHAP-based interpretable diagnostic framework for alzheimer's disease. *BMC medical informatics and decision making, 23*(1), 137.
96. Loveleen, G., Mohan, B., Shikhar, B. S., Nz, J., Shorfuzzaman, M., & Masud, M. (2023). Explanation-driven HCI model to examine the mini-mental state for Alzheimer's disease. *ACM Transactions on Multimedia Computing, Communications and Applications, 20*(2), 1–16.
97. Rashmi, U., Singh T., & Ambesange, S. (2023). MRI image-based ensemble voting classifier for Alzheimers disease classification with explainable AI technique. *2023 IEEE 8th international conference for convergence in technology (I2CT)*, Lonavla, India, pp. 1–6, https://doi.org/10.1109/I2CT57861.2023.10126269.
98. Viswan, V., Shaffi, N., Mahmud, M., Subramanian, K., & Hajamohideen, F. (2024). Explainable artificial intelligence in Alzheimer's disease classification: A systematic review. *Cognitive Computation, 16*(1), 1–44.
99. Hasan Saif, F., Al-Andoli, M. N., & Bejuri, W. M. Y. W. (2024). Explainable AI for Alzheimer detection: A review of current methods and applications. *Applied Sciences, 14*(22), 10121.
100. Shen, S., Han, S. X., Aberle, D. R., Bui, A. A., & Hsu, W. (2019). An interpretable deep hierarchical semantic convolutional neural network for lung nodule malignancy classification. *Expert Systems with Applications, 128*, 84–95.
101. Kumar, D., Sankar, V., Clausi, D., Taylor, G. W., & Wong, A. (2019). Sisc: End-to-end interpretable discovery radiomics-driven lung cancer prediction via stacked interpretable sequencing cells. *IEEE Access, 7*, 145444–145454.

102. Xi, P., Shu, C., & Goubran, R. (2018, June). Abnormality detection in mammography using deep convolutional neural networks. In *2018 IEEE international symposium on medical measurements and applications (MeMeA)* (pp. 1–6). IEEE.
103. Windisch, P., Weber, P., Fürweger, C., Ehret, F., Kufeld, M., Zwahlen, D., & Muacevic, A. (2020). Implementation of model explainability for a basic brain tumor detection using convolutional neural networks on MRI slices. *Neuroradiology, 62*, 1515–1518.
104. Yang, X., Wang, Z., Liu, C., Le, H. M., Chen, J., Cheng, K. T., & Wang, L. (2017). Joint detection and diagnosis of prostate cancer in multi-parametric MRI based on multimodal convolutional neural networks. In *Medical image computing and computer assisted intervention–MICCAI 2017: 20th international conference, Quebec City, QC, Canada, September 11–13, 2017, proceedings, Part III 20* (pp. 426–434). Springer International Publishing.
105. Gulum, M. A., Trombley, C. M., & Kantardzic, M. (2021). Multiple interpretations improve deep learning transparency for prostate lesion detection. In *Heterogeneous data management, polystores, and analytics for healthcare: VLDB workshops, poly 2020 and DMAH 2020, virtual event, august 31 and September 4, 2020, Revised Selected Papers 6* (pp. 120–137). Springer International Publishing.
106. Venugopal, V. K., Vaidhya, K., Murugavel, M., Chunduru, A., Mahajan, V., Vaidya, S., Mahra, D., Rangasai, A., & Mahajan, H. (2020). Unboxing AI-radiological insights into a deep neural network for lung nodule characterization. *Academic Radiology, 27*(1), 88–95.
107. Zhen, S. H., Cheng, M., Tao, Y. B., Wang, Y. F., Juengpanich, S., Jiang, Z. Y., Jiang, Y. K., Yan, Y. Y., Lu, W., Lue, J. M., & Cai, X. J. (2020). Deep learning for accurate diagnosis of liver tumor based on magnetic resonance imaging and clinical data. *Frontiers in Oncology, 10*, 680.
108. Wang, C. J., Hamm, C. A., Savic, L. J., Ferrante, M., Schobert, I., Schlachter, T., Lin, M., Weinreb, J. C., Duncan, J. S., Chapiro, J., & Letzen, B. (2019). Deep learning for liver tumor diagnosis part II: convolutional neural network interpretation using radiologic imaging features. *European Radiology, 29*, 3348–3357.
109. Papanastasopoulos, Z., Samala, R. K., Chan, H. P., Hadjiiski, L., Paramagul, C., Helvie, M. A., & Neal, C. H. (2020, March). Explainable AI for medical imaging: deep-learning CNN ensemble for classification of estrogen receptor status from breast MRI. In *Medical imaging 2020: Computer-aided diagnosis* (vol. 11314, pp. 228–235). SPIE.
110. Afshar, P., Plataniotis, K. N., & Mohammadi, A. (2019, September). Capsule networks' interpretability for brain tumor classification via radiomics analyses. In *2019 IEEE international conference on image processing (ICIP)* (pp. 3816–3820). IEEE.
111. LaLonde, R., Torigian, D., & Bagci, U. (2020). Encoding visual attributes in capsules for explainable medical diagnoses. In *Medical image computing and computer assisted intervention–MICCAI 2020: 23rd international conference, Lima, Peru, October 4–8, 2020, Proceedings, Part I 23* (pp. 294–304). Springer International Publishing.
112. Pintelas, E., Liaskos, M., Livieris, I. E., Kotsiantis, S., & Pintelas, P. (2020). Explainable machine learning framework for image classification problems: Case study on glioma cancer prediction. *Journal of Imaging, 6*(6), 37.
113. Blendowski, M., & Heinrich, M. P. (2019, May). Learning interpretable multi-modal features for alignment with supervised iterative descent. In *International conference on medical imaging with deep learning* (pp. 73–83). PMLR.
114. Munshi, R. M., Cascone, L., Alturki, N., Saidani, O., Alshardan, A., & Umer, M. (2024). A novel approach for breast cancer detection using optimized ensemble learning framework and XAI. *Image and Vision Computing, 142*, Article 104910.
115. Wani, N. A., Kumar, R., & Bedi, J. (2024). DeepXplainer: An interpretable deep learning based approach for lung cancer detection using explainable artificial intelligence. *Computer Methods and Programs in Biomedicine, 243*, Article 107879.
116. Silva-Aravena, F., Núñez Delafuente, H., Gutiérrez-Bahamondes, J. H., & Morales, J. (2023). A hybrid algorithm of ML and XAI to prevent breast cancer: A strategy to support decision making. *Cancers, 15*(9), 2443.

117. Singhal, A., Agrawal, K. K., Quezada, A., Aguiñaga, A. R., Jiménez, S., & Yadav, S. P. (2024). Explainable artificial intelligence (XAI) model for cancer image classification. *CMES-Computer Modeling in Engineering & Sciences, 141*(1).
118. Khater, T., Hussain, A., Mahmoud, S., & Yasen, S. (2023, December). Explainable AI for breast cancer detection: A LIME-Driven approach. In *2023 16th international conference on developments in eSystems engineering (DeSE)* (pp. 540–545). IEEE.
119. Nitha, V. R., & SS, V. C. (2025). An explainable machine learning framework for predicting the impact of pesticide exposure in lung cancer prognosis. *Journal of Computational Science, 84*, 102476.
120. Cimino, M. G., Campisi, G., Galatolo, F. A., Neri, P., Tozzo, P., Parola, M., ... & Di Fede, O. (2025). Explainable screening of oral cancer via deep learning and case-based reasoning. *Smart Health*, 100538.
121. Hauser, K., Kurz, A., Haggenmüller, S., Maron, R. C., von Kalle, C., Utikal, J. S., Meier, F., Hobelsberger, S., Gellrich, F. F., Sergon, M., Hauschild, A., … & Brinker, T. J. (2022). Explainable artificial intelligence in skin cancer recognition: A systematic review. *European Journal of Cancer, 167*, 54–69.
122. Ghasemi, A., Hashtarkhani, S., Schwartz, D. L., & Shaban-Nejad, A. (2024). Explainable artificial intelligence in breast cancer detection and risk prediction: A systematic scoping review. *Cancer Innovation, 3*(5), Article e136.
123. Karthiga, R., Narasimhan, K., & Amirtharajan, R. (2024). Review of AI & XAI-based breast cancer diagnosis methods using various imaging modalities. *Multimedia Tools and Applications*, 1–52.
124. GhoshRoy, D., Alvi, P. A., & Santosh, K. C. (2023, March). Unboxing industry-standard AI models for male fertility prediction with SHAP. In *Healthcare* (vol. 11, No. 7, p. 929). MDPI.
125. GhoshRoy, D., Alvi, P. A., & Santosh, K. C. (2022). Explainable AI to predict male fertility using extreme gradient boosting algorithm with SMOTE. *Electronics, 12*(1), 15.
126. Xu, F., Ma, Q., Lai, P., Hu, L., Gao, C., Xu, Q., Fang, Y., Guo, Y., Yao, W., & Zhang, C. (2024). An explainable machine learning model based on ultrasound for predicting reproductive outcomes after frozen embryo transfer. *Reproductive BioMedicine Online*, 104743.
127. Lee, T., Natalwala, J., Chapple, V., & Liu, Y. (2024). A brief history of artificial intelligence embryo selection: From black-box to glass-box. *Human Reproduction, 39*(2), 285–292.
128. Mohammed, K., & Shehu, A. (2023). A review of artificial intelligence (Ai) challenges and future prospects of explainable AI in major fields: A case study of Nigeria. *Open Journal of Physical Science (ISSN: 2734–2123), 4*(1), 1–18.
129. Curchoe, C. L., Malmsten, J., Bormann, C., Shafiee, H., Farias, A. F. S., Mendizabal, G., Chavez-Badiola, A., Sigaras, A., Alshubbar, H., Chambost, J., Jacques, C., … Rosenwaks, Z. (2020). Predictive modeling in reproductive medicine: Where will the future of artificial intelligence research take us?. *Fertility and Sterility, 114*(5), 934–940.
130. Hanassab, S., Nelson, S. M., Akbarov, A., Yeung, A. C., Hramyka, A., Alhamwi, T., Salim, R., Comninos, A. N., Trew, G. H., Kelsey, T. W., Heinis, T., … Abbara, A. (2025). Explainable artificial intelligence to identify follicles that optimize clinical outcomes during assisted conception. *Nature Communications, 16*(1), 296.
131. Hanassab, S., Nelson, S. M., Akbarov, A., Yeung, A. C., Hramyka, A., Alhamwi, T., Salim, R., Comninos, A. N., Trew, G. H., Kelsey, T. W., Heinis, T., … Abbara, A. (2024). O-219 Explainable artificial intelligence (XAI) to determine the follicle sizes on trigger day that maximize mature oocyte yield. *Human Reproduction, 39*(Supplement_1), deae108–258.
132. Afnan, M. A. M., Liu, Y., Conitzer, V., Rudin, C., Mishra, A., Savulescu, J., & Afnan, M. (2021). Interpretable, not black-box, artificial intelligence should be used for embryo selection. *Human Reproduction Open, 2021*(4), hoab040.
133. Sharma, A., Stensen, M. H., Delbarre, E., Haugen, T. B., & Hammer, H. L. (2022, June). Explainable artificial intelligence for human embryo cell cleavage stages analysis. In *Proceedings of the 3rd ACM workshop on intelligent cross-data analysis and retrieval* (pp. 1–8).

134. Setegn, G. M., & Dejene, B. E. (2024). Explainable artificial intelligence models for predicting pregnancy termination among reproductive-aged women in six east African countries: Machine learning approach. *BMC Pregnancy and Childbirth, 24*(1), 600.
135. Luong, T. M. T., Ho, N. T., Hwu, Y. M., Lin, S. Y., Ho, J. Y. P., Wang, R. S., Lee, Y. X., Tan, S. J., Lee, Y. R., Huang, Y. L., Hsu, Y. C., … Tzeng, C. R. (2024). Beyond black-box models: explainable AI for embryo ploidy prediction and patient-centric consultation. *Journal of Assisted Reproduction and Genetics, 41*(9), 2349–2358.
136. Nwokoro, C. O., Inyang, U. G., Eyoh, I. J., Umoh, U. A., Duke, O. A., Nwokoro, K. C., Opara, P. I., Obinachi, C., & Kingsley, J. U. (2023). Enhancing maternal outcome prediction using explainable artificial intelligence for women of childbearing age. *Asian Journal of Science and Applied Technology, 12*(2), 44–55.
137. Rahman, A., & Alam, M. G. R. (2023, June). Explainable AI based maternal health risk prediction using machine learning and deep learning. In *2023 IEEE World AI IoT Congress (AIIoT)* (pp. 0013–0018). IEEE.
138. Valencia, R., Farías, A. F. S., Mendizabal, G., Chavez-Badiola, A., & Gomez, F. J. A. (2022). Towards an explainable artificial intelligence to predict blastocyst formation potential from single oocyte images. *Fertility and Sterility, 118*(4), e337–e338.
139. Kebede, S. D., Abera, K. M., Abeje, E. T., Bekele Enyew, E., Daba, C., Asmare, L., Demeke Bayou, F., Arefaynie, M., Mohammed, A., Tareke, A. A., Keleb, A., Kebede, N., Tsega, Y., & Endawkie, A. (2024). Explainable machine learning for modeling predictors of unintended pregnancy among married/in-union women in sub-Saharan Africa, a multi-country analysis of MICS 6 survey. *Digital Health, 10*, 20552076241292976. https://doi.org/10.1177/20552076241292978
140. Jain, P., Mishra, R. K., Deep, A., & Jain, N. K. (2024). Xplainable AI for deep learning model on PCOD analysis. In *XAI Based Intelligent Systems for Society 5.0* (pp. 131–152). Elsevier.
141. Çiçek, İB., Küçükakçalı, Z., & Yağın, F. H. (2021). Detection of risk factors of PCOS patients with local interpretable model-agnostic explanations (LIME) method that an explainable artificial intelligence model. *The Journal of Cognitive Systems, 6*(2), 59–63.
142. Moral, P., Mustafi, D., & Sahana, S. K. (2024). PODBoost: An explainable AI model for polycystic ovarian syndrome detection using grey wolf-based feature selection approach. *Neural Computing and Applications, 36*(30), 18627–18644.
143. Khanna, V. V., Chadaga, K., Sampathila, N., Prabhu, S., Bhandage, V., & Hegde, G. K. (2023). A distinctive explainable machine learning framework for detection of polycystic ovary syndrome. *Applied System Innovation, 6*(2), 32.
144. Dewanjee, S., Muntaha, S., & Uddin, M. N. An XAI-Integrated BiLSTM-GRU-CNN framework for early polycystic ovary syndrome detection.
145. Mahesswari, G. U., & Maheswari, P. U. SmartScanPCOS: A feature-driven approach to cutting-edge prediction of polycystic ovary syndrome using machine learning and explainable artificial intelligence.
146. Elmannai, H., El-Rashidy, N., Mashal, I., Alohali, M. A., Farag, S., El-Sappagh, S., & Saleh, H. (2023). Polycystic ovary syndrome detection machine learning model based on optimized feature selection and explainable artificial intelligence. *Diagnostics, 13*(8), 1506.

Chapter 6
Summary and Take-Home Messages

This chapter serves as a summary of the book, offering key take-home messages drawn primarily from the author's own experiences. It is not intended to be an exhaustive review, but rather a reflective synthesis that highlights the most practical insights and lessons learned throughout the journey presented in the preceding chapters.

In Chap. 1, we comprehensively examined the relationship between human fertility and global dynamics, using the Total Fertility Rate (TFR) as a key indicator. Through this lens, we analyze global metrics such as population growth, Gross Domestic Product (GDP), and the Human Development Index (HDI). The discussion encompasses critical factors including economic development, educational empowerment, family planning and healthcare services, cultural influences, environmental conditions, urbanization, global migration, and population aging, providing a nuanced understanding of fertility's pivotal role in national and global economies. To achieve these insights, we adopted a multifaceted approach. First, we investigated how TFR impacts population metrics and its correlation with GDP, HDI, and other social factors. For the initial analysis, we utilized datasets from *Our World in Data* and the *United Nations Population Fund*. This revealed the top five countries with the highest TFR—Niger, Chad, Somalia, the Democratic Republic of Congo, and the Central African Republic—and examined the underlying factors contributing to these elevated rates. Graphical analyses illustrated the relationship between global TFR and that of high-TFR countries. Comparative assessments between developed nations and the global average further provided context to current fertility trends. Additionally, an overview of population growth rates was presented, along with strategic recommendations to address declining birth rates in developed economies. The second section of the chapter focuses on the relationship between GDP and TFR, highlighting how economic performance and fertility are interconnected. By categorizing 141 countries into six geographic regions—Western Europe and related nations, Eastern Europe, Asia, Latin America and the Caribbean, Arab States, and Sub-Saharan Africa—the study revealed distinct patterns. A visual analysis of GDP and TFR across these regions demonstrated that countries with lower fertility rates

KC. Santosh and D. G. Roy, *Artificial Intelligence for Human Fertility: Trends, Insights, and Predictions*, Studies in Computational Intelligence 1230,
https://doi.org/10.1007/978-981-95-1248-5_6

consistently exhibit higher GDP per capita than regions with elevated TFRs, emphasizing the economic implications of fertility trends. In the third analysis, the correlation between HDI and TFR is explored. The comparison of the top 10 countries with the highest HDI and their fertility rates to the top 10 with the lowest HDI demonstrated a clear inverse relationship: as HDI increases, TFR tends to decrease. This observation underlines the strong linkage between human development and fertility behaviour, suggesting that nations with higher development indices are more likely to experience lower fertility rates. The final section addresses the influence of social factors on fertility rates, considering elements such as religiosity, family structures, marital trends, and education. The analysis highlights the significant impact of religious beliefs on fertility patterns and notes a transition in family systems, which plays a crucial role in shaping fertility trends. Furthermore, the study reveals the intricate relationship between marital practices and fertility rates, reinforcing the role of sociocultural norms in demographic trends.

In Chap. 2, we explored human reproductive dynamics with a specific focus on key reproductive determinants. Two primary indicators, Crude Birth Rate (CBR) and Total Fertility Rate (TFR), form the foundation of this analysis. Initial observations examine trends in TFR and CBR among the ten most populous countries, revealing that in seven of these nations, the TFR falls below the replacement level. To enhance the precision of the study, Age-Specific Fertility Rate (ASFR) is incorporated, offering a more nuanced understanding of global reproductive trends. Drawing on data from diverse sources such as DHS, NS, and UNSD, this study investigates the interplay between TFR, CBR, ASFR, and the mean age of childbearing. The analysis identifies notable contrasts, such as the low TFR observed in China and the high-TFR reported in Nigeria, reflecting significant variations in reproductive dynamics across nations. Further exploration into infertility prevalence among the world's top ten most populous countries sheds light on the broader implications and underlying causes of reproductive challenges, creating a comprehensive framework for understanding reproductive health determinants. Human reproduction is examined holistically in this chapter, encompassing physical, mental, and social dimensions. Male-specific factors influencing reproduction include hormonal dysfunction, physical conditions, sexual disorders, lifestyle influences, environmental exposures, and genetic or epigenetic anomalies. Female-specific factors encompass ovulatory disorders, endometriosis, pelvic adhesions, tubal blockages, uterine abnormalities, and hyperprolactinemia. Additionally, certain factors impair reproductive health in both genders, such as age, medication use, illicit drug consumption, obesity, substance abuse, occupational exposures, psychological stress, and levels of physical activity. The chapter also emphasizes the importance of prevention and management strategies for reproductive health issues, particularly those related to infertility, conception, and pregnancy. Infertility poses widespread socio-economic and psychological consequences, often resulting in stigma, depression, and diminished overall well-being. To address these challenges, lifestyle modifications are highlighted as critical preventive measures, including improvements in diet, increased physical activity, and stress reduction. Education and awareness about reproductive health also play a vital role in fostering informed decision-making. Diagnostics, such as clinical assessments, laboratory testing, and imaging, are discussed as essential tools for accurately evaluating reproductive health. Non-invasive and invasive treatment protocols are outlined, offering effective solutions to improve reproductive outcomes. The involvement of healthcare professionals is emphasized as a cornerstone of successful prevention, diagnosis, and treatment efforts. A multidisciplinary approach is essential for addressing the complexities of reproductive health challenges. This analysis underscores the interconnectedness of reproductive health with broader determinants of physical, mental, and social well-being. Implementing targeted strategies and evidence-based practices offers significant opportunities to improve reproductive health outcomes, address challenges related to infertility, and foster overall societal well-being.

In Chap. 3, we presented an in-depth and expansive examination of artificial intelligence and its transformative potential in the healthcare domain. It begins with a comprehensive introduction to the evolving role of AI in modern healthcare systems, emphasizing how AI technologies are increasingly being integrated into critical areas such as medical imaging interpretation, remote and digital consultations, predictive analytics for disease progression, clinical decision support systems, surgical and assistive robotics, remote patient monitoring, electronic health record analysis, personalized medicine, administrative automation, disease diagnosis, and the drug discovery pipeline. Following this introduction, the chapter outlines the fundamentals of AI models and their operational workflows that underpin healthcare applications. It emphasizes the importance of structured workflows in AI model development, including data acquisition, preprocessing, model training, validation, deployment, and continuous monitoring. Critical factors influencing the performance and feasibility of AI systems are explored in detail, such as the availability and quality of healthcare datasets, the computational resources required for training and inference, algorithm tuning strategies, cost-efficiency considerations, the need for specialized infrastructure or laboratory setups, clinical interpretability of features, and the broader limitations and ethical concerns surrounding the deployment of AI in clinical environments. A central component of the chapter is devoted to feature engineering, which encompasses feature selection, feature extraction, and data handling techniques. Both traditional and contemporary feature selection methods are discussed in depth, including Correlation-Based Feature Selection, consistency-based filtering, interaction-based approaches, information gain, Relief algorithms, and Recursive Feature Elimination. The strengths and limitations of each method are compared, along with guidance on selecting appropriate techniques based on specific problem types, dataset characteristics, and clinical objectives. In contrast, various types of feature extraction methods are presented, categorized into linear and nonlinear approaches, along with their objectives and application contexts. Linear techniques such as Principal Component Analysis, Linear Discriminant Analysis, Independent Component Analysis, Singular Value Decomposition, and Non-negative Matrix Factorization are discussed alongside nonlinear approaches including Kernel PCA, autoencoders, t-distributed Stochastic Neighbour Embedding, Isomap, Uniform Manifold Approximation and Projection, Locally Linear Embedding, Laplacian

Eigenmaps, and Multidimensional Scaling, with a focus on their performance implications in clinical data analysis. The chapter also provides a structured overview of various AI algorithms commonly used in healthcare analytics. These include traditional machine learning techniques such as decision trees, support vector machines, k-nearest neighbours, and logistic regression, as well as ensemble learning models like random forests, gradient boosting, and stacking methods. The advantages of ensemble approaches in improving predictive accuracy, reducing model variance, and enhancing generalizability are highlighted. The conceptual relevance of these algorithms is linked to practical healthcare scenarios, where accurate predictions and reliable decision support are critical. Overall, this chapter synthesizes the theoretical foundations, methodological approaches, and applied strategies of AI in healthcare, offering a valuable resource for researchers, clinicians, and developers. It underscores the importance of interdisciplinary collaboration and continuous innovation in harnessing the full potential of AI to transform healthcare delivery and medical research.

In Chap. 4, we provided an in-depth exploration of the role of artificial intelligence in reproductive medicine. It begins by outlining the advantages of AI over conventional methods, emphasizing its potential to enhance diagnostic accuracy and decision-making. The discussion then transitions to the use of AI in assessing human fertility, focusing on key contributing factors. These include lifestyle, behavioural habits, obesity, age, and genetic predispositions—all of which play a significant role in reproductive health. The chapter examines how AI models leverage these features to generate predictive insights, representing a major advancement in fertility research. A dedicated section explores the application of medical imaging in fertility prediction. Specific indicators such as ovarian functionality, follicle development, and polycystic ovary syndrome detection are highlighted. These factors are primarily related to female reproductive health and offer critical information for early diagnosis. The methodology segment introduces contemporary techniques in dimensionality reduction and data balancing, along with their impact on AI model performance and reliability. Subsequently, the chapter discusses commonly used AI algorithms, including Decision Tree, Support Vector Machine, Convolutional Neural Networks, Artificial Neural Networks, Naïve Bayes, K-Nearest Neighbours, Random Forests, XGBoost, and Logistic Regression. Each algorithm is examined in terms of its applications, strengths, limitations, and notable use cases within reproductive medicine. The chapter also features a comprehensive review of case studies, divided into two main sections. The first focuses on male fertility assessment, particularly sperm morphology and semen quality, which are essential parameters for evaluating male reproductive potential. A variety of studies demonstrate that AI-based methods often outperform traditional approaches in these areas. Multiple algorithms have been employed to assess sperm morphology, and semen quality predictions have been significantly enhanced with AI-based techniques. Furthermore, we describe how AI-enabled systems offer improvements over standard laboratory-based semen analysis. The second section examines female fertility assessment using AI. It highlights various strategies for diagnosing conditions such as PCOS, which affects an estimated 105 million women globally, and endometriosis, a leading cause of infertility affecting approximately 190 million women worldwide. These conditions are frequently underdiagnosed through conventional means. Additional focus is given to uterine fibroids and primary ovarian insufficiency. Many AI-driven approaches have shown promise in detecting these issues at early stages, providing faster, more accessible, and less invasive alternatives to traditional diagnostic procedures. Despite these technological strides, the application of AI in female fertility remains constrained, primarily due to the limited availability of large, diverse datasets. In the concluding section, we present conceptual insights emphasizing that AI model development is still evolving. Creating robust and reliable models requires meticulous feature selection, appropriate algorithm choice, and rigorous external validation. Although both traditional and ensemble methods yield encouraging results, determining their optimal use remains a key challenge. In addition, the widespread adoption of AI in reproductive healthcare is hindered by several significant challenges. These include the limited availability of comprehensive datasets, the often-opaque nature of AI model decision-making, and the hesitation among clinicians to move away from established medical guidelines. As a result, effective integration of AI into reproductive medicine requires strong collaboration between AI specialists and healthcare professionals. Such cooperation is essential to build trust, enhance the interpretability and usability of AI systems, and ensure that these technologies align with clinical needs and standards.

In Chap. 5, we discussed on role of Explainable Artificial Intelligence (XAI) in healthcare, with a particular focus on reproductive medicine, which holds significant promise. This chapter examines the potential applications of XAI, the methodologies for its implementation, and its critical importance in advancing healthcare systems. A comprehensive overview of various XAI methods and their corresponding strategies underscores their utility in addressing complex challenges in medical domains. The discussion begins with an outline of the stages where XAI can be applied and categorizes the methods into six distinct types: feature-oriented techniques, global techniques, concept models, surrogate models, local methods, pixel-based approaches, and human-centric techniques. These methodologies are explored in depth to highlight their operational scope and effectiveness. Additionally, seven prominent XAI tools—AI Fairness 360, What-If Tools, Skater, H2O platform, SHAP, ELI5, and Distill—are analyzed in terms of their developers, sources, purposes, and technical specifications. Once XAI systems are deployed, rigorous evaluation becomes imperative. This work details evaluation schemes, emphasizing both objective and subjective metrics, and illustrates their importance with examples from real-world applications. Such evaluations ensure the reliability, interpretability, and effectiveness of these systems. The discussion expands to encompass the application of XAI across multiple healthcare domains. Existing literature emphasizes the role of XAI in promoting the transparency and usability of AI systems, thereby facilitating acceptance among clinicians, healthcare professionals, and the public. By simplifying complex AI processes and enhancing trustworthiness, XAI enables a more seamless integration of AI into clinical and operational settings. Beyond reproductive medicine, XAI demonstrates immense potential in addressing critical health issues, such as cancer, Alzheimer's disease, and cardiovascular disease (CVD). Cardiovascular disease, being a leading cause of mortality, affects millions worldwide, while cancer continues to exert an increasing societal burden, with annual patient numbers rising. Alzheimer's disease disrupts individual lives and social structures and ranks as the sixth leading cause of death. These conditions also exhibit close associations with fertility-related health concerns and comorbidities. For instance, studies suggest that a woman's reproductive history may influence her risk of developing Alzheimer's, while cancer treatments often lead to fertility challenges. Similarly, infertility in men has been linked to a higher likelihood of cardiovascular diseases. In this context, XAI offers critical insights to interpret and address these interrelated health challenges. Within the realm of reproductive medicine, XAI's applications extend far beyond fertility assessments. It provides transformative insights into areas such as improving in vitro fertilization (IVF) outcomes, supporting gamete selection, diagnosing polycystic ovary syndrome, evaluating childbearing risks, advancing male fertility diagnostics, and enhancing maternal health. These contributions reinforce XAI's critical role in supporting and advancing human reproductive health. The review of case studies reveals that XAI represents an emerging and rapidly developing research area. Researchers are increasingly recognizing its transformative potential, particularly in reproductive medicine. The concluding analysis underscores the urgent need for greater attention to implementing XAI in this field, as it holds the potential to drive innovation and improve healthcare outcomes comprehensively.

In brief, here is our take-home message: Infertility is an increasingly prevalent global issue, affecting approximately 48.5 million couples. However, unlike other major health conditions such as cardiovascular diseases, chronic pulmonary disease, Alzheimer's disease, diabetes, and cancer—each receiving substantial attention for their widespread impact—infertility remains comparatively overlooked. Despite its significant prevalence, infertility is often underestimated as a health concern due to its lack of clear symptoms and is typically diagnosed only when individuals struggle to achieve parenthood. This delayed recognition frequently leads to considerable emotional, financial, and psychological strain. Many individuals, after investing substantial resources and hope, may face failure, which results in dissatisfaction, stress, and social stigma. Furthermore, discussions surrounding reproductive health remain taboo in many societies, limiting data availability and impeding efforts to effectively address infertility. The lack of awareness about infertility's societal and economic implications, particularly its impact on national growth and development, exacerbates the issue.

In this context, AI emerges as a transformative tool. AI can serve as a clinical support system, assisting physicians in identifying factors contributing to infertility on an individual basis. This is especially valuable in regions with limited medical infrastructure, insufficient clinicians, and inadequate diagnostic resources. AI-driven systems facilitate early diagnosis, reducing both time and costs. While clinicians often prescribe numerous diagnostic tests that impose significant financial burdens on patients, AI has the potential to enhance primary healthcare systems, thereby mitigating these challenges. However, the adoption of AI in clinical settings faces hurdles due to its perceived complexity. To address this, Explainable AI (XAI) has been introduced. XAI increases the transparency of AI systems by clarifying how specific features influence decision-making processes, fostering greater acceptance and accountability within the medical field, including reproductive healthcare. In addition, assisted reproductive technologies such as in vitro fertilization, intracytoplasmic sperm injection, and intrauterine insemination play a crucial role in supporting parenthood for infertile couples. These techniques offer hope; they are probabilistic, do not guarantee success, and often impose significant financial burdens. With the integration of AI, clinicians can better predict the likelihood of successful pregnancies, thereby alleviating emotional stress and reducing financial strain on patients.

A significant gap exists in research and published literature on reproductive health, underscoring its status as an undervalued global issue. Data scarcity, often due to restrictions imposed by authors or institutions, poses another critical challenge. Addressing infertility as a major health concern is essential for the holistic development of nations. Individual awareness, coupled with a willingness to share data, is vital to advancing reproductive healthcare systems worldwide.

MIX
Papier aus verantwortungsvollen Quellen
Paper from responsible sources
FSC® C105338

If you have any concerns about our products,
you can contact us on
ProductSafety@springernature.com

In case Publisher is established outside the EU,
the EU authorized representative is:
Springer Nature Customer Service Center GmbH
Europaplatz 3, 69115 Heidelberg, Germany

Printed by Libri Plureos GmbH
in Hamburg, Germany